NAVIGATING YOUR HOSPITAL STAY

A Guide Written By Expert Nurses

Editors: Mary Beth Modic, DNP, APRN, CNS, CDE &
Christina Marie Canfield, MSN, APRN, ACNS-BC, CCRN-E

ISBN (Print) 978-1-48359-293-0 (Ebook) 978-1-48359-294-7

Editors Mary Beth Modic and Christina Canfield

Sponsored by treasury funds from the Stanley Shalom Zielony Institute for Nursing Excellence

Front cover image by Helen D'Souza
Cleveland Clinic Main Campus photographs by Yu Kwan Lee

Printed in USA
First Printing February 2017
Published by BookBaby
7905 N Crescent Blvd
Pennsauken, NJ 08110

TABLE OF CONTENTS

Part Three:
Partnering with your Caregivers to Manage
Your Chronic Medical Conditions 143

Part Four:
Partnering with Your Caregivers when You Require Surgery 265

Part Five:
Partnering with Your Caregivers
in the Care of Special Populations 303

Foreword

K. Kelly Hancock, DNP, RN, NE-BC

I f you have ever had a loved one admitted to the hospital, you know first-hand how much you rely on the nurses and doctors to answer your questions, keep you informed and provide state-of-the-art care. If you have been hospitalized, you know the questions that ran through your mind when you were being admitted: Will I be all right? How long will I be in the hospital? Who is going to take care of me? You may have been concerned about being in pain, being away from your family, being able to sleep or having to ask hospital staff for help. These questions and fears are very real and are shared by most people being admitted to the hospital.

This book was written by expert nurses who want to help you and your loved ones prepare for a hospital stay. Clinical Nurse Specialists at Cleveland Clinic have included important information that will help you to recover and stay informed while in the hospital. The Clinical Nurse Specialists who have written this book are some of the most experienced and educated nurses working in hospitals today. Their wisdom and experience have helped thousands of patients overcome their fear of being in the hospital, recover from their illnesses or surgeries and prepare for discharge. From the cradle to the end of life, in the lives of many, there is no reliable substitute for a nurse. We want to help you through your hospital experience, and we will be there right beside you.

This book describes the members of the caregiving team you or your loved one may encounter, the role of the bedside nurse and why care is provided in certain ways. The goal of this book is to help you become an educated partner in your hospital stay or that of your loved one. The messages contained in this book encourage you to speak up, ask questions and offer feedback to your caregivers.

During your hospital stay, you are the most important member of the caregiving team. Being an active partner in your care or your loved one's care will help you get the right treatment, right information and right discharge plan. There is a lot to do and learn while you are in the hospital besides healing from your illness or surgery. You will need to know and understand the plan for discharge, the best way to regain your strength and energy and what activities will help you get better and stay safe.

While being an active partner and standing up for yourself is extremely important, know that you won't be the only one trying to protect your or your loved one's best interests. The caregiving team will also be looking out for you, as well as speaking up for you. A registered nurse will be assigned to care for you and oversee your care 24 hours a day. Your nurse will take your vital signs, give you medications and monitor your response to treatments. Your nurse will listen to your worries, fears and anxieties. Your nurse will communicate these concerns to other members of the caregiving team. Your nurse will ease your suffering and protect you from harm. Your nurse will keep you informed about your progress. Your nurse will help you reduce the chances for complications from your illness or surgery. Your nurse will teach you about your medications and how to manage your symptoms at home. Your nurse will help you rest and comfort your loved ones. Your nurse is committed to your well-being and healing.

Patients and their loved ones are the reason hospitals exists. Providing safe, compassionate and expert care is the overarching goal of your doctors, nurses and other caregivers in the hospital. I hope you will use this book as a guide to help you through your hospital stay. It will provide you with the questions you should be able to answer before you or your loved one is discharged. It will explain the role of each member of the caregiving team so that you know what to expect. It will offer resources that you can use to learn more about your illness or help you cope. The book should convey the message that YOU are the important member of the caregiving team.

Preface

Florence Nightingale, the founder of modern nursing, was also a social reformer. Because of her dedication to the soldiers, diligent record keeping and political savviness, she was able to publicize the horrific conditions of British soldiers serving in the Crimean War that were contributing to their deaths. She was also responsible for bringing to light the dreadful conditions in military hospitals and was integral in redesigning them so that they were clean and spacious and provided fresh air, warmth, quiet and ample light. In addition to improving hospitals, Florence Nightingale also created the first pharmacy, nutrition service, laundry, infection control processes and patient library. She also created the first school of nursing in London that bears her name. She was unrelenting in her pursuit of excellence, new knowledge and continuous improvement.

What would Florence Nightingale say about nursing in the 21st century and the quality of care that is provided in hospitals? We think she would be amazed with all of the technological advances, scientific discoveries and innovative therapies available to cure disease, alleviate suffering and extend the lifespan. We also think that she would remind us to remain vigilant, proactive and patient and family-centered.

The authors of this book are expert nurses who have achieved clinical excellence caring for patients throughout the lifespan. Each has experienced being admitted to a hospital and sitting at the bedside of a loved one. We have marveled at the skill and compassion of caregivers and have also been frustrated by the gaps in and coordination of care. We were able to advocate for ourselves and our loved ones because we are nurses and knew how to consult with our colleagues to get the information we were desperately seeking and have our concerns addressed. But what if you are not a nurse, physician or hospital executive? How do you navigate the complexity of a hospital stay?

In discussing our experiences, it was suggested that a book should be written by nurses to educate patients and their loved ones. The purpose of this book is to provide you with important information about what to expect when you or a loved one is admitted to the hospital and how to advocate when the experience is not what you anticipated, wanted or needed.

This book is organized into five sections:

Section 1: "Introducing You to the Hospital Environment" describes the process of being admitted to the hospital, knowing your rights and responsibilities as a patient, interacting with the different caregivers who will be providing care and participating in your plan of care. It also contains information about using technology to become an informed and empowered patient. In addition, this section emphasizes the importance of partnering with your caregivers so you can communicate your needs, wants and preferences.

Section 2: "Identifying Nursing Care Practices: Comfort, Safety and Education" highlights the care that is provided by the bedside nurses assigned to care for you. The nurse's role in evaluating and monitoring your response to medication and treatments are described. Intentional safety practices – including protecting you against infections and preventing falls, medications errors and pressure ulcers – are also discussed. This sections provides important information on how bedside nurses advocate, teach and protect you while you are in the hospital and prepare you to be discharged.

Section 3: "Partnering with Your Caregivers to Manage Your Chronic Medical Condition" contains important information about common chronic medical conditions that are associated with frequent hospitalizations. A detailed list of questions you should be able to answer in order to self-manage your illness confidently at home is presented at the end of each chapter. Websites that contain accurate and reliable information to assist you in the day-to-day decision making of living with your illness are also included.

Section 4: "Partnering with Your Caregivers when You Require Surgery" answers frequently asked questions about the surgical experience, most importantly how to reduce potential complications and recover quickly. This section also provides recommendations to help you manage after discharge from the hospital. The book describes the care of frequently performed surgical procedures, not all surgeries are included.

Section 5: "Partnering with Your Caregivers in the Care of Special Populations" addresses the differing and unique care needs of the very fragile neonate and older adult to the laboring woman. It also offers strategies on how to advocate for children, those that are disabled and those suffering from Alzheimer's. The nurse experts will speak to the distinct needs of each of these special groups.

Your nurses and doctors recognize the capability of you and your loved ones and want you to feel heard, validated and respected as you describe your fears, needs and expectations. Florence Nightingale understood this idea well when she wrote in *Notes on Nursing: What it is and What it is Not* in 1860, "Apprehension, uncertainty, waiting, expectation, fear of surprise do more harm than any exertion." It is our hope that this book will encourage and enable you to be a full partner in your hospital care.

Mary Beth Modic, DNP, APRN, CNS, CDE Christina Canfield, MSN, APRN, ACNS-BC, CCRN-E

Acknowledgements

The final stanza from "Oh the Places You'll Go" by Dr. Seuss is "So... be your name Buxbaum, or Bixby or Bray or Mordecai Ali Van Allen O'Shea' you're off to Great Places! Today is your day! Your mountain is waiting. So... *get on your way!* " Our book idea would have gone nowhere without the encouragement, expertise, and enthusiasm of so many.

We are indebted to Kelly Hancock, Chief Nurse Executive of the Cleveland Clinic Health System and Chief Nursing Officer of Cleveland Clinic Main Campus, for her unwavering support of the writing of this book. Dr. Hancock has been integral to enhancing the experience of patients, promoting the practice of nursing and encouraging nursing research and innovation. Without her encouragement, our book would have been lost.

We are grateful to Meredith Lahl, Associate Chief Nursing Officer of Advanced Practice Nursing, for her guidance. She spent many hours removing the road blocks which emerged in trying to get our book published. Without her direction, we would have been off course.

We appreciate the hundreds of patients who offered feedback about the content of this book. Their thoughtful comments and recommendations provided us with the navigational tools to let us know that we were on the right path. Special thanks to Scott Steele, Manager of Market Research and Innovations at Cleveland Clinic for his skill in soliciting patient feedback and collating their valuable suggestions. He was our "GPS".

We would like to thank Mandy Barney, Project Manager for the Cleveland Clinic Zielony Nursing Institute who served as navigator for the writing of the book. She brought the book to its destination – publication!

We are thankful for the skill of Yu Kwan Lee, a gifted photographer, for visually capturing the important work of nurses. We also appreciate the work of other members of the Art and Photography Department who prepared the photos for publication. Their work enriched the journey.

We appreciate the artistry of Helen D'Souza who created the cover for our book. Her captivating illustrations reflect the thinking, caring and healing practices of nurses everywhere. Her beautiful compass captured the message we wanted to convey – nurses represent the hands and hearts of healthcare and are central to the provision of safe and high quality care. She was the "way finder" of our message.

We would like to acknowledge with great affection and respect, our nursing colleagues at Cleveland Clinic who shared their clinical wisdom, expertise and time in authoring chapters for the book. They are remarkable men and women whose intellect, compassion and skill make a difference in the lives of patients and their loved ones every day. They scrutinized the literature so they could share the most current and best evidence to support their recommendations. They sojourned with us. They made getting to the "mountain top" possible.

Mary Beth Modic

I wish to express my profound gratitude to my colleagues in the Center for Excellence in Healthcare Communication, Ms. Jessica Crowe and Drs. Katie Neuendorf, Rich Frankel, Tim Gilligan, Rachel Taliercio, V.J. Velez and Amy Windover. Their passion for modeling, teaching and promoting relationship centered care is simply extraordinary. I am so very fortunate to work with these dedicated, empathic and brilliant individuals. They showed me the way to the "mountain top" and what a road map they shared!

Last, but never least, I want to acknowledge my loving family who provide the compass for everything I do. To my husband, Mark, our children Anna, Mark, Josie, Daniel, Stefan and Claire, their spouses, Andrew, Jessie and Dave, and grandchildren, Emerson, Jack, Beatriz, Reese, Emery and Louise I say thank you. Of all the places, I have ever gone and may go in the future, being with them will always be my favorite place. "It is for you that my heart beats."

Christina Canfield

I would like to extend the deepest gratitude to my colleagues Catherine Skowronsky, Julie Simon and Dianna Copley. These amazing individuals play an important role in my life as my sounding board, my support and my professional consultants. They work tirelessly to make the world better for nurses and the patients for whom they care. I am fortunate to not only call them colleagues, but friends.

I would also like to acknowledge and thank my family for their support through the development of this book. My husband Curt, son Matthew and daughter Meredith are always there at the end of the day to support and encourage.

Part One:

Introducing You to the Hospital Environment

"The first requirement in a hospital is that it should do the sick no harm"
-Florence Nightingale

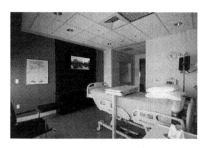
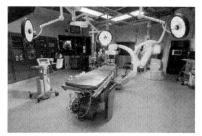
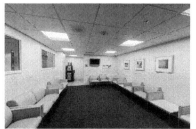
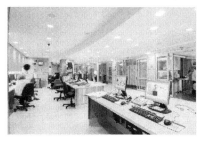

Being Admitted to the Hospital

Mary Beth Modic, Christina Canfield, Christian Burchill

Whether your admission was planned or unexpected, being admitted to the hospital is very unsettling. It may appear chaotic if the admission is unplanned. You may be admitted because of a sudden medical illness or traumatic injury. You may be transferred from another hospital or nursing home because you require a higher level of care. Your admission may be planned because of a scheduled surgery. However you are admitted, your condition will direct the intensity and pace of the interactions you have with the individuals who will be taking care of you.

How will I know if I need to be admitted to the hospital?

You may be admitted to the hospital if your medical condition becomes worse – you have difficulty breathing, unstable vital signs (such as a high or low blood pressure or pulse), pain that is unrelieved by over-the-counter or prescribed pain relievers, abnormal laboratory findings or change in level of consciousness.

Most of the time, the reason is known and your doctor has a clear idea of what is needed to resolve or minimize your condition. Occasionally, symptoms may be vague or unusual and 24-hour monitoring and diagnostic testing that cannot be performed as an outpatient are necessary to identify the diagnosis. Specific questions that you would want to ask your doctor about being admitted to the hospital include:

- "Why do I need to be admitted?"
- "What is my diagnosis?"
- "How long do you expect I will need to stay in the hospital?"
- "What tests or treatments will I need?"
- "What are the risks if I choose not to be admitted to the hospital?"
- "Are there other options to treating my condition without being admitted?"

Who will be caring for me?

Many hospitals have adopted the term "caregiver" to refer to all the individuals with whom you and your loved ones will interact. This term encompasses all of the healthcare professionals who will provide direct care to you as well as all of the ancillary and "behind the scenes" individuals who influence the quality and safety of your hospital experience. Caregiver will be the term used in this book when referring to any healthcare professional or ancillary personnel.

If there is a specific caregiver who is responsible for a certain aspect of your care – doctor, nurse, pharmacist, dietician, for example – those individuals will be referred to by their professional role. The term healthcare provider will be used to describe the person who is responsible for monitoring your overall health. It could be a doctor, nurse practitioner, nurse midwife or physician assistant. This individual evaluates your response to the treatment plan.

What information will my caregivers need to know about me?

Your doctors and nurses will ask questions about your general health, current health problem, family history, past hospitalizations and surgeries, social history and current medications you are taking. You may begin to feel like everybody is asking you the same questions. In many cases, this is necessary to gain additional perspectives on how to best take care of you. It is important that you be as honest and accurate as possible as your treatment plan will be based on your answers. Be forthcoming about medication that you often forget to take or prescriptions that were never filled. This will prevent your doctor from making treatment decisions based on inaccurate information, such as ordering a higher dose of a medication, believing that your previously prescribed dose is not working.

You may experience many emotions while you are in the hospital. Worry, fear and anxiety are very common. You may also feel helpless, vulnerable or experience a loss of control as you depend on others to help you with bathing, eating or toileting needs. You may feel confused because of the number of people caring for you or as a result of conflicting information that is provided to you. You may feel anger if your care does not meet your needs or expectations. You may also feel a sense of panic, denial or hopelessness because of the shock of a devastating or unanticipated diagnosis. It is important to share these feelings with your doctors and nurses so that they can tailor their care to meet your individual needs and coping styles.

What should I bring to the hospital?

Because you may be hospitalized for an extended stay, you're encouraged to bring whatever will help you feel comfortable. Some suggestions:

- Personal identification and emergency contact information
- All cards that contain insurance information
- A copy of your advance directives – "living will" and "durable power of attorney for healthcare"
- A current list of medications, including over the counter and herbal supplements
- Glasses, contacts and hearing aids
- Dentures and denture care products

- Cane, walker or any other device that helps or physically supports you as you walk. Be sure each item is labeled with your name and address.
- Cell phone and charger. Hospitals permit the use of cell phones in certain areas.
- Toiletries. Although the hospital usually provides these items, you may wish to bring your own personal toiletry products, including deodorant.
- Notepad and pen (helpful for remembering questions to ask your caregiving team). It might be helpful to bring a zip-top storage bag for business cards and other paperwork received during your stay. This way the information you collect can be stored in one location.
- Sweat pants, t-shirts, robe, slippers and pajamas. Loose, comfortable clothing if you expect your hospital stay to be lengthy. Loose clothing provides access for the medical equipment that might be needed for daily physical assessment.
- Your favorite music on your smartphone or tablet
- Family pictures or other reminders of home

What items should I leave at home?

Although it is helpful to have a list of the medications and dosages that you take at home, it is not necessary to bring your medications with you. Any medication you currently take at home will be provided by the hospital pharmacy during your stay. It is very useful to your caregivers if you write down the name and dosage of all of your medications and bring the list with you.

Please avoid bringing to the hospital the following items:

- Jewelry
- Credit cards, checks, large amounts of cash
- Firearms or weapons of any kind

If you want to bring your valuable electronic equipment, such as a laptop or tablet, check with the hospital to see if they have a safe available for use.

Refrain from wearing artificial nails or nail polish since these items can interfere with monitoring your oxygen levels.

How often can my family and friends visit me?

Having family and friends visit can be very comforting and reassuring. It is a good idea to think ahead about having your family and friends visit at different times while you are in the hospital so that you are not over-whelmed with company. You might want to ask others to call ahead to see if you feel up to a visit. It is important to remember that you are recovering from surgery or a severe illness and you need to rest and not feel obligated to entertain your visitors. Although visiting hours may be flexible, it's recommended to limit the number of visitors at one time and to observe reasonable hours.

Visiting a sick parent can be traumatic for children if they are unprepared for the change in physical appearance, mood or energy level. It is important to discuss with other family members how best to prepare children for a visit. It is also wise to check with your bedside nurse as to when it would be best for your children to visit and how your nurse can orient your child to the equipment. It is very important that your child feel safe in your presence and not be worried about you, so it is best to have your child visit when your pain is under control and energy level may be somewhat normal.

All visitors should wash their hands before entering your room, and sick visitors should refrain from visiting. Usually patient bathrooms are only for patients. Public restrooms are available for visitor use and are usually equipped with diaper changing tables for babies. Check with your bedside nurse if you have questions about children or overnight visitors.

How will my family be updated?

We know that there are many people who are concerned about you. It is difficult for the caregiving team to speak to several members of your family about your progress at different times. For this reason, most hospitals request that the patient identify one spokesperson to whom information will be provided. In most situations, your spokesperson is the individual who holds your durable power of attorney for healthcare. Sometimes it is best to deliver information in a planned meeting of selected family and friends. This is called a family meeting and allows for questions and concerns to be discussed in a group setting. A family meeting usually involves the physician, nurse, social worker and a chaplain. If you or your loved ones believe that there are differing opinions between you, your family and members of the caregiving team, share your concerns with your nurse so a meeting may be arranged.

The Health Insurance Portability and Accountability Act of 1996 prevents caregivers from discussing the care and status of patients in the hospital with anyone other than the patient. As a result, when family members call in to speak with the nurse for an update, it may be frustrating that this information cannot be provided over the phone. Check with your nurse to determine what will be the best way for you to be kept informed of your loved one's condition. Some hospitals use codes or passwords to identify individuals who may be provided with updates.

How often will someone check on me?

The frequency of monitoring will depend on the acuity of your illness or condition. If your vital signs are unstable, you will be admitted to the Intensive Care Unit (ICU) where a registered nurse will continuously monitor you. There will be nurses, physicians and respiratory therapists in the ICU 24 hours a day.

Outside of the ICU, your monitoring will be less frequent. Your bedside nurse will be the caregiver who will spend the most time with you. Your bedside nurse will work with your nursing assistant to check on you at least every hour around the clock. Your nurse or nursing assistant will also check on when you put on your "nurse call light." On hourly rounds, your nurse will evaluate your vital signs and physical comfort, administer medications and intravenous (IV) fluids and perform treatments such as dressing changes. Your nurse will attend to subtle changes in your clinical condition and inform your doctor of significant changes. Your nurse will also engage you in conversation to assess your response to treatments and medications, as well as your emotional wellbeing.

Your attending physician will visit you at least once a day. In the hospital, caregivers refer to the doctor's visit as "making rounds." Your doctor and residents (if admitted to a teaching hospital) may make very quick rounds in the early morning to physically check in on you and then will return later to discuss your progress and the plan for your continued care. This is the time to ask your doctor questions you have about your condition, treatment or medications. Your bedside nurse, a pharmacist, a case manager and resident doctors may also be included in the rounds. Consultant physicians will also visit routinely until they no longer need to be involved in your care.

If you or one of your loved ones think that your condition is deteriorating or that something is "not right," please contact your nurse immediately. If your concerns regarding your symptoms are not being heard or acknowledged, you may activate the Rapid Response Team (RRT). The RRT is a team of caregivers usually comprising a physician, nurse and respiratory therapist who respond to patients outside of the ICU to assess patients and prevent further decline.

Examples of urgent conditions include:

- Unresolved anxiety or a feeling that something just isn't right
- Sudden changes in your breathing rate or breathing pattern
- Change in mental status – confusion, loss of orientation (name, date, place)
- Increased or sudden chest pain
- Uncontrolled pain in any part of your body

Information on how to contact the Rapid Response Team is usually included in your admission packet or on a handout on your bed stand in your hospital room. If this information is not provided to you on admission, please ask your bedside nurse.

This chapter has concentrated on what you can expect when you are admitted to the hospital. It includes recommendations for what you should bring to the hospital and what you should leave at home. It also describes ways in which you and your family will be updated about your progress and how frequently a member of the caregiving team will be checking on you. Being knowledgeable about hospital practices will help you be an active participant in your care.

Being Admitted to the Hospital via the Emergency Department

Karen Guzi

I f you are being admitted to the hospital from the emergency department (ED), chances are you are feeling very ill or have been injured in an accident. You may be in pain, feeling stressed or becoming impatient. The ED can be a busy place. The national average for wait times is four hours. The purpose of this chapter is to help explain what influences ED wait times and what you can expect from your visit in the ED.

What items should I bring to the emergency department?

If you or your loved one is seriously ill or injured, you will probably be quite anxious. It may be challenging to remember important information that the doctors and nurses will want to know. Documents that contain important health information should be brought to the ED. These include:

- List of prescriptions
- List of allergies
- List of illnesses or medical conditions
- Driver's license or identification card

- Medical insurance card

List of emergency contacts with phone numbers. (This information may be important to the caregiving team so that they will know whom to contact in the event that you would be unable to communicate.)

Prepare these lists in advance before an emergency, and keep an updated copy in your wallet or purse.

How do caregivers decide the order in which patients will be seen?

Patients are not seen in order of arrival, but rather how ill they are when they come through the ED doors. Each patient who presents to the ED has his or her condition evaluated and is triaged according to the seriousness of the illness or injury. The registered nurse will ask questions about when your illness started, what other symptoms you are having and the type of pain you are experiencing. The nurse will also take your vital signs (pulse, blood pressure, temperature, respiratory rate and sometimes oxygen saturation level) to assist in determining the severity of your condition.

How long does treatment take?

If it is determined that you are seriously ill, you will be moved quickly to an examining room where treatment, diagnostic procedures and medications will be administered. If your illness or injury is life-threatening, it may take many hours to stabilize your condition. Once you are stabilized, you will be admitted to the hospital for further monitoring, treatment and evaluation.

If you are presenting to the ED without a life-threatening illness – such as sore throat, ear ache, minor cut in which bleeding has stopped or a chronic condition in which the symptoms have persisted for several weeks – your wait could exceed four hours. Going to the ED for non-medical emergencies increases the time you must wait to be seen.

Is there a time to go the ED when I will be seen more quickly?

Emergency departments get busier in the afternoon and during flu season.

Can my family stay with me while I am in the emergency department?

In most cases, even in the most emergent situations, your family or close friends may stay with you. Your caregivers may ask your visitors to step out during procedures or when you are being examined. If you wish for some privacy, please ask your visitors to take a break or request that your caregivers limit visitation.

Why am I being asked the same questions by different caregivers?

While many hospital emergency departments use a computerized medical record to hold all of your health data, there may be times when different caregivers ask you the same question. This can be frustrating, but necessary. You may remember to tell the nurse something that you forgot to tell the doctor. Your answers to the questions can help the members of the caregiving team best determine which tests or treatments are necessary.

How will my pain be managed in the emergency department?

Your caregiving team appreciates that pain relief is important when someone is hurt or needs medical attention. Every effort will be made to treat your acute pain so that you are comfortable. You will be asked to describe your pain including the location, intensity/severity, how long you have had it, and anything you have done or taken to treat it. Providing an accurate description of your pain can be very helpful to your caregiving team.

Managing pain in a patient in the ED is challenging. This is because misuse of pain medication can cause serious health problems. In the ED, narcotic pain medication is only prescribed for acute pain. If you are discharged from the ED, pain medication with the lowest possibility of addiction and overdose will be prescribed.

What can I do to prevent getting an infection while I am in the hospital?

Proper hand hygiene is to be performed by all caregivers, either by hand washing with soap and water or use of alcohol foam/gel. Caregivers are to wash their hands upon entering the room, when gloves are removed and upon exiting the room. Caregivers should also wash with soap and water if their hands become visibly soiled during care. Hand hygiene is one of the most important practices to prevent the spread of infection. It is OK and strongly encouraged to remind any caregiver to perform hand hygiene at any time.

How do I know that the nurses are giving me the right medication given the busyness of the ED?

Hospitals have put safety practices in place to prevent medication errors. Patient identity is verified before any medication is given or any treatment or procedure is performed. Patients are asked to state their name and date of birth. Another verification practice performed by nurses is to compare the information on their patients' wristbands with information located in the computer.

Another safety practice is the use of a barcode scanning program to assist with accurate medication administration. Your identification wristband has a unique barcode that will be scanned before any medication is given. The information encoded in the barcode allows for the comparison of medication being administered with what is in the medication record. Barcode medication administration systems are designed to prevent medication errors in healthcare settings and improve the quality and safety of medication administration. Barcode medication administration may be used in all areas of the hospital.

Can I eat while I am in the emergency department?

Patients in the emergency department are generally not permitted to eat or drink until the cause of the illness or extent of injuries is determined. Caregivers may use the term "NPO," which means nothing by mouth (from Latin, nil per os). Once all of your tests or diagnostic studies are completed, your caregivers will decide if it is safe for you to eat or drink. If the answer is yes, you may be offered something to drink or a small snack.

What happens if I need to be admitted to an observation unit?

You may need additional monitoring beyond what can be provided in the emergency department. Observation or Clinical Decision Units (CDU) provide an alternative for patients not ill enough to be admitted to the hospital, but not well enough to be discharged home. Some of the common conditions for admission to an observation unit include chest pain, atrial fibrillation, heart failure, asthma, back pain and dehydration. A patient's stay in an observation or decision unit lasts less than 24 hours. Patients are either discharged or admitted as inpatients to the hospital after this time.

What should I keep with me when I am admitted to the hospital?

Once you are admitted to the hospital, there will be no need to keep the medications you take at home with you in the hospital. Please send them home with your loved ones. Your nurse will make a list of all of the belongings you keep with you. Keep your eyeglasses, hearing aids, dentures and walking aids. Please ask your nurse to label your cane or walker with your name, if it is not labeled before you are admitted. Before you are transferred from the ED to your inpatient room, be sure all of your belongings are with you.

This chapter has focused on what you can expect when you visit the Emergency Department. It includes suggestions for what you should bring to the hospital and what you should expect about waiting if you do not have a life- threatening illness or injury. It also answers frequently asked questions (FAQs) about the ED experience.

Knowing Your Rights and Responsibilities

Mary Beth Modic

The American Hospital Association (AHA) is an organization that represents hospitals, healthcare systems, their patients and communities. This organization has created a document to guide hospitals in creating partnerships between caregivers and patients. Each hospital has established unique patient rights and responsibility statements that reflect their organizational mission, vision and values.

The rights and responsibilities of patients described below address major themes. When you are admitted to the hospital you have rights as a patient.

What are my rights as a patient?

You have the right to:

- **High-quality patient experience** – Your care should be patient centered, designed to meet your physical, emotional and spiritual needs. All of your caregivers should provide expert, respectful and compassionate care. Each caregiver should communicate clearly and answer your questions so that you understand the plan of care

– what is being done and why – and what you can do to aid in your recovery. All caregivers should identify themselves by their name, discipline and license. You have the right to know if the caregiver is a student or resident physician. "I am Dr. John Foster. I am a 3rd year medical resident. I will be working with Dr. Kate McBride, who is your attending physician." "My name is Marcia Harris, and I am your registered nurse who will be taking care of you today." "I am the physical therapist who will be working with you today. My name is Jose Santiago." You have the right to request a change in caregiver or request a second opinion.

- **Clean and safe environment** – Providing safe care to patients is a priority for all hospitals. Hospital executives have made the prevention of infections and medical errors a priority. Creating physical environments that are comforting, healing and provide privacy have also received a great deal of attention. The Joint Commission, an organization that surveys and accredits hospitals and other healthcare organizations for quality and safety practices, has established the following safety goals:

  ✓ Identify each patient correctly
  ✓ Communicate with other caregivers effectively
  ✓ Use medicines safely
  ✓ Use alarms correctly
  ✓ Prevent infections
  ✓ Identify patients at risk for injury
  ✓ Prevent mistakes in surgery

- **Involvement in your care** – Your caregivers want you to speak up when you have questions or do not understand the tests, treatments or procedures that have been ordered to treat your condition. The risks and benefits of all procedures and operations need to be explained to you so that you may consent with a complete understanding of the need and outcome of the procedure. If any explanation is unclear, please ask for further clarification. If one of your caregivers appears distracted or impatient when interacting with you, ask when your question or concern can be fully addressed. Do not be intimidated by a caregiver who is aloof, disengaged or condescending. It is important that you feel respected, acknowledged and valued by all caregivers.

- **Protection of your privacy** – Your caregivers value the importance of privacy and will work diligently to provide it and protect it. Every hospital has written policies about how personal and health information is protected.

- **Preparation for discharge** – During your hospital stay, your nurse will evaluate your home going needs. Along with your doctor, your nurse will discuss with you and your loved ones whether you will be able to manage at home or whether you will need additional nursing care. Referrals may be made to a case manager or social worker. Instructions about new medications, activity, treatments, diet, new treatments and any symptoms that warrant a call to your doctor will be provided before you leave the hospital.

- **Information about your hospital bill/ insurance forms** – Reading hospital bills and completing insurance forms can be very complicated. Personnel in hospital billing offices are available to provide explanations about your bill.

What are my responsibilities as a patient?

It is your responsibility to do the following:

- **Provide accurate and reliable information about your overall health** – Identify the reason(s) you are seeking medical attention, any past illnesses, hospitalizations and surgeries. Bring a list of prescribed and over-the-counter medications that you take regularly. Offer an explanation for the medications that are problematic for you, whether it be side effects, cost or frequency of dose. Sharing your "story" will help your caregivers individualize your care.

- **Make your physical needs known** – Share any change in your physical condition with your caregiver right away. This will allow your nurse and doctor to address the problem right away before any symptom gets worse. Some examples of a change in condition include a sudden increase in pain, difficulty breathing or an inability to urinate.

- **Make your personal and cultural needs known**-these may be related to your ethnic heritage, belief patterns, religion, preferred name, gender identification or sexual orientation.

- **Speak up** – Ask questions when an explanation is unclear. Ask for assistance when you need or want it. Share worries and concerns. All of your caregivers are dedicated to alleviating your pain, suffering and anxiety. This can only occur when you verbalize your needs or fears. You are the expert on you!

Expressing your expectations to your caregivers will assist them in developing a plan that will help you recover more quickly. Your caregiver team should be providing daily updates (at a minimum). If you or your loved ones are not being informed of your progress, ask to speak with your admitting doctor. The Joint Commission has created a Speak Up ™ initiative with brochures, videos and infographics that encourage patients to take a more active role in their healthcare. The information includes questions to ask your caregivers and describes what you and your loved one should expect. Speak Up™ materials can be accessed from the JCAHO website: http://www.jointcommission.org/facts_about_speak_up_initiatives/

- **Follow the instructions provided by your caregivers** – Your recovery depends on your willingness and ability to participate in your treatment. It is very important to take your medications and take an active role in your therapies as prescribed. If you have concerns about your medications or feel that you are unable to participate in your therapies, share these with your bedside nurse. Your caregiving team, most especially your doctors and bedside nurses, want you to recover and heal. Medications, food, activity, rest and therapies help you to do this. If there are obstacles in your life that will prevent you from purchasing your medications or following a prescribed diet due to cost, lack of social support or transportation, you need to share these obstacles with your doctors and nurses. Medications can be changed and other ways of getting you to follow up appointments and care can be arranged.

Statements of patient rights and responsibilities are posted in different locations throughout each hospital and may be available on their websites. Some hospitals may provide written statements of your rights and responsibilities when you are admitted. It is a good idea to review these statements when making healthcare choices.

What is meant by the term "Patient Experience"?

Caregivers have come to the conclusion that providing excellent clinical care is not enough to satisfy patients and their loved ones. Patients want to be seen as individuals and to know that their caregivers care about them. They want their caregivers to be approachable and empathic and to acknowledge their suffering, fears and anxieties. Patients want their caregivers to deliver on their promises. Patients also want to understand the instructions caregivers provide and want their caregivers to appreciate the obstacles they may encounter in following the prescribed treatment.

Although there is no consensus definition for patient experience in the healthcare literature, most caregivers would agree that a positive patient experience requires highly skilled, compassionate and thoughtful caregivers who provide safe and quality care in a respectful, efficient and timely manner.

Examples of caregiver behaviors that contribute to a positive "patient experience" include:

- Greeting you by your preferred name
- Introducing themselves to you and your loved ones
- Including your loved ones in conversations about your care (if that is your desire)
- Attending to your personal privacy
- Treating you with dignity and respect
- Listening deeply to your worries, fears and concerns
- Comforting you when you are distressed
- Conveying an appreciation of the meaning and magnitude your illness has on you and your loved ones
- Providing clear explanations so you can make informed decisions
- Keeping you and your loved ones informed of your progress
- Collaborating with you in creating the plan of care
- Accepting questions/challenges from you and your loved ones about treatments, medications and other care decisions graciously
- Teaching you about your medications and self-care practices for managing your health at home
- Confirming your understanding of the discharge and follow-up plan

What do I do if my expectations are not being met by my caregivers?

This chapter has concentrated on what you can expect when you are admitted to the hospital. Establishing a relationship with your caregivers will help in having your expectations met. If you have concerns or questions, share these with your bedside nurse. If you believe that your concerns remain unaddressed, ask to speak to the nurse manager. The nurse manager or assistant nurse manager visit patients frequently to identify any issues patients and their loved ones have with their care. They are grateful when patients share their dissatisfaction or disappointment with their care while they are in the hospital so that the issues can be addressed right away.

Also, tell your attending physician so that he or she has the opportunity to correct the situation. If your concern is with your attending physician, remember that you have a right to consult with another physician. You may also seek out assistance from a member of the Ombudsman Department. Individuals from this department are skilled in resolving differences between caregivers and patients.

What websites could I use to learn about the quality of care that is provided at my hospital?

There are many organizations that collect and report information about quality of care and patient satisfaction. This information is readily available on the Internet. Listed below are a few organizations that provide information about overall quality.

American Hospital Association
www.heart.org

Joint Commission
http://www.jointcommission.org

Medicare Hospital Compare
http://www.medicare.gov/hospitalcompare

The Leapfrog Group
http://www.leapfroggroup.org

Recognizing Members of your Healthcare Team

Mary Beth Modic & Christina Canfield

When you are admitted to the hospital there is an ensemble of individuals who will be directing, planning and providing expert care to you. These individuals will communicate with each other and will inform you and your loved ones about your progress. They will also discuss any procedures or diagnostic tests that may be needed to help you recover. It is important to know the names of each of your caregivers and their role in your recovery and healing.

Who are the individuals who will be taking care of me?

Your team of caregivers may include the following physicians, nurses and other caregivers:

Physicians

Physician: Physician is the term used to distinguish those who practice medicine from dentists, podiatrists, optometrists and psychologists. A physician is an individual who is a graduate of an accredited medical school. Some physicians are licensed as Medical Doctors (M.D.). Others are licensed as Doctors of Osteopathy (D.O.), depending on where they received their medical education. The course of study is four years after college. An internship, residency and fellowship are required to specialize and sub-specialize. Residencies can range from three to seven years or more of supervised medical training depending on the specialty.

Attending/Staff Physician: This physician has assumed primary responsibility for your care. The attending physician will be the individual who directs your care, assesses your progress and determines if other specialists are required to assist in addressing your medical needs.

Fellow: A Fellow is a physician who has completed the basic residency program and is concentrating on a specific specialty. A Fellow is a senior physician member of the team.

Resident: A Resident is a physician who is completing different clinical rotations to acquire the skills necessary to complete medical training.

Intern: An intern is a physician who has completed medical school and is in the first year of postgraduate training. An intern is often referred to as a first-year resident.

Consultant Physician: This physician specializes in an area of medicine other than your admitting physician. Examples include physicians who specialize in care of patients with infections, diabetes, breathing problems, foot ulcers and depression.

Hospitalists: These are physicians who are employed by the hospital and whose primary clinical focus is the general medical care of hospitalized patients. Their activities include patient care, teaching, research and leadership related to hospital medicine. The Hospitalist manages the care of the patient only while the patient is hospitalized.

Surgeon: A surgeon is a physician who specializes in the performance of surgery. Surgeons **determine** the diagnosis and provide care before, during and after an operation.

Nurses

Registered Nurse (RN): A registered nurse is an individual who is a graduate of an accredited nursing program. The course of study ranges from two years to four years and beyond. Nurses are the caregivers who have the most direct contact with you during your hospital stay. A Registered Nurse is assigned to care for you 24 hours a day while you are in the hospital.

Clinical Nurse: This registered nurse, also referred to "bedside" nurse in this book, is responsible for planning and coordinating your care with other members of the caregiver team. This individual will provide 24-hour monitoring to determine how well you are progressing and recovering from your illness. Your bedside nurse will administer medications and evaluate how well they are working. Your bedside nurse will also teach you about what you need to do when you get home to continue your recovery. This Registered Nurse will be the link to your physicians and all other caregivers.

Licensed Practical /Vocational Nurse (LPN/LVN): This nurse has completed a one-year program of study and is a graduate of an accredited practical/vocational program. The licensed practical/vocational nurse works in collaboration with the registered nurse to provide your care.

Nursing Assistant (NA): The nursing assistant is an unlicensed individual who has received specialized training in performing activities of daily living such as bathing, toileting, walking and taking vital signs. The Nursing Assistant works under the direction of the RN.

Nurse Manager: The nurse manager oversees the nursing staff, which includes the RNs, LPNs, nursing assistants and the unit coordinators. The nurse manager is the administrator for the nursing unit and ensures the quality and safety of the care that is provided. The nurse manager collaborates with all of the physicians involved with your care.

Assistant Nurse Manager: The assistant nurse manager assists the nurse manager in "round the clock" operations of the nursing unit.

Case Manager: The case manager is a registered nurse or social worker who identifies healthcare needs, living arrangements and social support for patients with complex social and financial needs. The case manager will work closely with you, your bedside nurse and your physician to determine the best arrangements for you once you leave the hospital.

Advanced Practice Registered Nurses

Nurse Practitioner (NP): The nurse practitioner is an advanced practice registered nurse who is a graduate of a master's or doctoral program in nursing. The nurse practitioner is licensed to prescribe medications and treatments. In addition, NPs can perform highly technical procedures for which they have received specialized training. The NP and attending physician collaborate closely on your plan of care.

Clinical Nurse Specialist (CNS): The clinical nurse specialist is an advanced practice registered nurse who is a graduate of a master's or doctoral program. The CNS is an expert in all facets of nursing care: direct care, teaching and research. They are often asked to see patients who have complex needs. Some CNSs are also licensed to order tests, treatments and medications.

Certified Nurse Midwife (CNM): The certified nurse midwife is an advanced practice registered nurse who is a graduate of a master's or doctoral program. The CNM is an expert in providing care during pregnancy and delivery. CNMs provide general women's healthcare throughout her lifespan. This care includes general health check-ups and physical exams, as well as prenatal, birth and postpartum care.

Certified Registered Nurse Anesthetist (CRNA): The certified registered nurse anesthetist is an advanced practice registered nurse who is a graduate of a master's or doctoral program. The CRNA is an expert in providing anesthesia to patients for undergoing all types of surgeries or procedures.

Other Healthcare Professionals and Caregivers:

Child Life Specialist: Child life specialists complete a four year program of study and must be professionally certified. Child life Specialists are experts in child development. They promote effective coping through a variety of activities such as play, education, music and art. They are also involved in the preparation of children who will be hospitalized. Child life specialists provide emotional support for families facing difficult circumstances.

Dietitian (RD/LD): Registered dietitians are experts in food and healthy eating. Clinical dietitians are licensed and have completed a four year degree in nutrition or a related field of study. In the hospital setting, dietitians are focused on the prevention and identification of malnutrition. They create menus and strategies to help you follow a medical diet as well as provide education about healthy eating. Clinical dietitians are consulted to provide expert recommendations when patients cannot take food by mouth.

Environmental Service Worker: Environmental service workers are individuals who take great pride in creating an environment that is safe, clean and comfortable for patients, their loved ones and their caregivers. Environmental service workers handle general cleaning tasks and are responsible for cleaning facilities to hospital standards. Environmental service workers are concerned about your well-being and are happy to modify your room to address your needs.

Lactation Consultant: Lactation consultants are registered nurses who work with you and your baby on breastfeeding positions and proper "latching on". They also assist in solving breastfeeding challenges.

Occupational Therapists (OT): Certified occupational therapists typically hold master's or doctoral degrees in occupational therapy from an accredited institution. They can provide treatments to help you recover or maintain daily living and work skills. Occupational therapists also provide care with individuals with developmental disabilities.

Ombudsman: Ombudsman are individuals who listen to patient and family complaints and attempt to resolve them by forwarding the concern to individuals who can address the problem. They are very skilled in helping patients "cut through the red tape" when patients believe their complaints are not being adequately addressed by their doctors, nurses or other caregivers.

Pastoral Care (Chaplain): Pastoral care providers offer spiritual care in the hospital. They offer spiritual counseling and emotional and spiritual support. They provide prayers, blessings, religious reading materials and contacts with local clergy. They may also function as healing services practitioners, who provide relaxation and stress management support through a variety of holistic modalities.

Patient Transporter: Patient transporters are individuals who are specially trained in the transfer of patients from one location to another. They are skilled in body mechanics and proper positioning as well as handling of equipment that you may require in your care.

Pharmacist (Pharm.D.): A pharmacist is the healthcare professional who is licensed to compound and dispense medications prescribed by physicians, dentists and advanced providers. A doctoral degree in pharmacy is now required to become a licensed pharmacist. Pharmacists complete two years of undergraduate study and four years in a College of Pharmacy. Pharmacists are concerned with all aspects of medication safety. Pharmacists review all medication orders for accuracy, potential interactions with other medications and indications for use. In some hospitals, pharmacists participate in rounds with the physicians and nurses, offering their expert opinion on the selection, dosage and timing of medications.

Phlebotomist: Phlebotomists are specially trained individuals who draw blood for diagnostic testing.

Physical Therapist (PT): A physical therapist is an individual who is a graduate of an accredited physical therapy program. A doctoral degree is now required to become a licensed physical therapist. The course of study is three years pre-professional study and three years of physical therapy education. PTs specialize in the assessment and treatment of various diagnoses that limit physical functioning. PTs may help you with mobility, endurance, range of motion, coordination, pain control and balance.

Physician Assistant (PA): Physician assistants are licensed and certified healthcare professionals who practice medicine in partnership with physicians. PAs complete a course of study that is generally two to three years in length. Physician assistants have a license to prescribe medications and medical treatments.

Respiratory Therapist (RT): A respiratory therapist is specially trained in assessing and treating conditions of the lungs. Respiratory therapists complete a course of training that is two to four years in length. Respiratory therapists may give you breathing treatments, inhalers or other therapies to improve your breathing.

Social Worker: Clinical social workers have earned a master's degree in social work. Clinical social workers help facilitate end of life care conversations and offer emotional support to frightened and fatigued family members. They also assist with the completion of legal documents such as a living will, healthcare power of attorney and advance directives. Social workers are experts in identifying resources that can assist those who have legal, financial or social concerns.

Speech Therapist: Speech therapists, also referred to as speech pathologists, assess, diagnose, treat and help to prevent communication and swallowing disorders. They will recommend an appropriate, safe diet and explain how to feed your loved one if there are special precautions. A Master's degree in speech pathology as well as state licensure is required to work as a speech therapist.

Unit Coordinator: The unit coordinator is an individual who functions as a liaison between the nursing staff and patients and their loved ones. This individual may answer call lights and assist with patient and family needs.

Volunteers: A volunteer is an individual who donates time to improve the experience of patients who are hospitalized. Volunteers may assist visitors with finding their way around the hospital. Some volunteers deliver mail to patient's rooms while others may spend time talking to or reading with patients.

This chapter has described the caregivers who may be involved in your care, their educational preparation and their role in your care. Each of your caregivers is committed to your wellbeing.

Ask them questions. Share your concerns. Partner with them in your care.

Participating in Your Plan of Care

Mary Beth Modic

The daily plan of care outlines the diagnostic tests, procedures and therapies that are being proposed to help identify your medical condition or evaluate your response to treatment. The plan of care is created at the time that you are admitted to the hospital and is evaluated and updated daily. Your inclusion in the plan of care is very important as is it allows you to be an informed and integral member of the caregiving team.

This chapter describes the components in the plan of care and its importance in delivering patient-centered care. The potential for communication breakdown will be described. Strategies you can use to be an informed, educated and empowered patient will also be presented.

What is included in my plan of care?

- Your primary diagnosis
- Planned tests
- Planned procedures
- Medication changes

- Nutritional changes
- Planned consults – physician, nutrition, physical, respiratory or social work
- Changes in treatment goals based on the patient's response to treatment
- Anticipated discharge date

Who is involved in deciding my plan of care?

Your attending physician will be the individual who will direct and oversee your care. Your attending physician will also determine if other specialists are needed to be brought in to assist in addressing your medical needs. If you are admitted to a teaching hospital your attending physician may check in on you with a number of other doctors, nurses and pharmacists.

You are the constant person on the caregiving team. Your doctors and nurses may change several times during your hospital stay so it is important that you or your loved ones be actively involved in deciding what you need in collaboration with your attending doctor.

How do I learn about my plan of care?

Before your doctor visits you, your progress or condition will have been reviewed and the results from tests and procedures will have been evaluated. A discussion will occur with the other members of the caregiving team about what therapies need to be changed, what therapies are effective and what can be discontinued. This information should be shared with you daily and will usually take place during "rounds" or when your doctor comes to check on you.

Why is a plan of care necessary?

A plan of care helps to ensure that all aspects of your physical, emotional, social and spiritual well-being are being addressed. It also reduces stress of the unknown, as you and your loved ones are kept informed and updated about your progress. The plan of care is the roadmap to your destination of discharge from the hospital.

Since there can be many people involved in your care, this is often where a breakdown in communication occurs. Disagreements about priorities in care can also result when there are multiple caregivers offering differing recommendations. There may also patient-doctor disagreement on several aspects of the plan of care.

Studies investigating how well patients and their loved ones understand the plan of care suggest that patient understanding is low. The lack of understanding can be a result of a patient's inability to comprehend the cause of his or her symptoms, limited understanding of the need or plans for diagnostic testing, difference in expectations and lack of knowledge regarding side effects of medications that have been administered.

How can I be sure I am included in the plan of care?

Know the names of the doctors, nurses, nursing assistants and other caregivers who are caring for you. Use the notepad you brought to the hospital with you to write their names down. You should know the name of your attending doctor – the doctor who is responsible for overseeing your care. Your attending doctor will be the caregiver who has the most accurate information about your needs, progress and plans for getting you discharged.

Write down questions that remain unanswered. Have this available when your attending doctor checks on you and updates you about your progress. You may also copy the personal care plan included at the end of this book to record your caregivers' names, scheduled tests and procedures, daily updates and issues that remain unresolved.

There have been national efforts directed at helping caregivers communicate more effectively. Educational offerings for caregivers have concentrated on helping doctors and nurses learn how to listen more intently, offer explanations more thoroughly and express empathy more frequently. Providing information that is meaningful and understandable to patients is the ultimate goal.

What should I do if I do not feel informed?

Share this concern with your attending doctor and your bedside nurse. Your doctor may think that you understand the plan. Information about your progress, necessary tests, new therapies and medications is usually shared with you (and your loved ones if you wish) when your doctor visits you. If you or your loved one is very ill many specialists may be involved in providing care. As a result, you may experience information overload or conflicting information. Your bedside nurses are the members of the caregiving team that spend the most time with you while in the hospital. They are great sources of information and can be the bridge between your doctors loved ones and you.

Communicating with you and your loved ones is a responsibility that your doctors and nurses take very seriously. Each of your caregivers want you to feel that you are informed and have been consulted in creating your plan of care. In many hospitals, white boards are attached to the wall across from the foot of the hospital bed and the names of your nurses and nursing assistants are listed. Tests, procedures and therapies for the day may also be posted. Other hospitals may use care plans that are printed from the information contained in your medical record, and this document is reviewed daily with you by your bedside nurse.

During "rounds" when your doctor comes to visit and checks on you, your attending doctor will want to hear from you. Your doctor will want to know how you are feeling, what are your worries and concerns and what questions you have. If you do not think this is happening, it is important to SPEAK UP. Your doctors and nurses want to make certain that you understand your plan of care. Being informed and being an active participant helps you to recover and heal more quickly.

Using Technology to be an Informed Patient

Marianela E. Iuppa

Information and technology are becoming an increasingly essential part of clinical care just as they play an important role in everyday life. These tools assist caregivers to make decisions, manage complex situations and receive alerts to deliver care more effectively and safely. Information is a comprehensive term that describes the collection and use of all the facts and figures captured by the machines and people in a clinical environment. Technology is the broad category for devices, their accessories, the processes by which they operate and their connections to other systems in order for these machines to store and synthesize information.

Why is information and technology so important for hospital stays?

The amount of information that you or your loved one receives during a hospital stay may be overwhelming. Your caregivers will provide explanations about the treatments they are performing. They will also present instructions on what you need to do to recover at home. They may also suggest websites or phone "apps" so that you may continue to learn about your condition in the comfort of your own home. Learning how to access health information is an essential skill whether you are a patient, family member or caregiver.

Today's healthcare environment requires many highly technical solutions to provide state of the art care that is safe and effective. Technology is powerful and provides a level of safety and communication necessary in today's digital environment. Harnessing these tools to work in the hospital so that they provide the essential monitoring and do not negatively impact the caregiver/patient relationship is very challenging.

Information

Why is understanding information so important to my care?

The American Medical Association (AMA) describes a person's ability to understand basic health information and use it to make appropriate healthcare decisions as health literacy. Health literacy has nothing to do with how smart a person is or how much schooling they have completed.

The Patient Protection and Affordable Care Act of 2010 defines health literacy as "the degree to which an individual has the capacity to obtain, communicate, process and understand basic health information and services to make appropriate health decisions." You need health literacy skills to:

- Locate information and healthcare services
- Communicate your needs and preferences to your healthcare providers or caregivers
- Determine the usefulness and meaning of the healthcare information provided
- Understand the choices and consequences of the healthcare recommendations and ramifications if you choose not to follow the treatment plan

Not understanding healthcare instructions can lead to:

- Taking the wrong amount of medication or taking too much or too little
- Using medical equipment incorrectly
- Being unaware of worsening symptoms and actions to take to manage them
- Seeking care before symptoms are life threatening
- Overlooking the importance of keeping follow-up appointments so health can be monitored
- Misunderstanding the importance of following up with another specialist
- Underappreciating the importance of eating healthfully, being physically active and getting enough sleep

All hospitals strive to produce accurate, reliable and understandable information for their patients and visitors. The more you understand the information you are given, the better prepared you are to help participate in your care and make informed decisions. It is equally as important for your caregivers to receive correct information from you because missing, incomplete or inaccurate information can contribute to miscommunications in care.

How can I protect my private medical information?

The Health Insurance Portability and Accountability Act of 1996 (HIPAA) Privacy Rule, a federal law, gives you rights to your health information and sets rules and limits on who can look at and receive your health information. The information that is protected under this law includes all information collected and stored in your medical record, billing and insurance information, conversations you have with caregivers and most other information that is collected and held for the purpose of providing your health care.

Despite hospitals best efforts to ensure information is locked down, information breaches can happen. There are several things that you can do to help ensure that your information is secure. You should know your rights related to accessing your own medical information. You should never disclose information to anyone who is not directly involved in your care. You should never provide information online unless through a secured site. For example, sending medical information in emails or text messages, or putting any health information on social networking pages or other types of intranet pages is not secure. Using computers at work or in public spaces to transmit health information is not recommended. You need to make sure personal computers and devices have the necessary security and passwords to protect any private information. Avoid taking pictures, video or any other type of digital recordings of your medical care.

What information am I able to view?

Under the HIPAA law, patients have a right to obtain copies of health information contained in their medical record. The information that can be requested is not limited to the medical record, but also includes information about your healthcare plan and payments that have been made. A copy of your medical record information is available by request. Requests are made through the medical records department in writing (a form is available to fill out, sign and date), and a processing fee may be required to obtain your records.

Maintaining accurate records is a shared responsibility between patients and caregivers. With so much information available, it becomes important to share necessary clinical data so that care is coordinated and consistent between hospitals, doctors' offices, retail pharmacies, laboratories, rehabilitation centers and many other locations where patients may receive care. For example, if you have struggled with high blood pressure over the years and your doctors have tried several different medications without success, it is essential for each new caregiver caring for you to know about your prior medication experiences so that a new plan of management can be identified.

How do I manage all the information given to me or my family during an admission?

One of the best techniques that patients and their families can use during a hospital admission is to keep all medical information handed to them in one location. A folder or a dedicated binder or envelope for all written information can help to keep information organized so that as questions come up you can reference these materials easily with your caregiving team. Additionally, many patients who are in the hospital for longer stays find that keeping a journal of who they have talked to and the topics discussed is useful when referring to information that was given verbally to them.

You will be given written information that summarizes the care that was provided to you and plans for future care. This paperwork is reviewed with you and your loved ones by your bedside nurse. It is very important that you and your loved ones ask questions if any of the instructions are unclear or differ from what you were previously told.

What are common terms used when discussing medical information?

- **PHI**: Protected health information is any information whether oral or recorded that could be used to identify an individual or health information about an individual. This information is protected by law under HIPAA.
- **HIPAA**: The Health Insurance Portability and Accountability Act (HIPAA) is a federal law that gives you rights to your health information and sets rules and limits on who can look at and receive your health information.

- **Social Networking**: Online service, platform, or site that focuses on facilitating the building of social relations among people through commonly shared links, information and terms.
- **Privacy**: The control over personal health information and the right not to divulge this information unless necessary in providing care. It is the confidentiality of information.
- **Security**: The administrative, physical and technical safeguards that are used to protect and store information. It is the measures taken to limit access to information.
- **Plan of care**: The set of actions that will be taken and the expected outcomes of these actions in order to resolve or support care that is provided to a patient, family, group or community.

Technology

What are the common types of technology used in hospitals?

Many different types of technology exist in hospitals today. These technologies are constantly changing to meet the increasing complexity of healthcare. Most equipment that nurses and doctors use come with a computer chip, wireless card or other form of computerized technology to help collect data and transmit information to other connected systems. Common examples of technology that are used every day that one might not think about include breathing machines (ventilators), IV pumps, wireless phones, patient call lights, patient beds, interactive televisions, barcoded wristbands, informational kiosk stations in lobbies, electronic medical records and digital cameras for skin and wound care.

What types of technology are used to care for me when I am admitted?

Patients often interact with technology throughout the course of their hospital stay. You may be asked to check in using tablet devices or waiting area computer kiosk stations. You may be asked to sign electronic consent forms using a signature pad similar to the types used in stores to collect credit card signature transactions. Your loved ones will be kept informed of your transitions in the operating room and when you have moved to the recovery room by an electronic messaging board.

Every time you have your blood pressure or temperature taken, the equipment collecting this data is all part of the suite of technology that caregivers commonly use to provide care. Perhaps one of the most important pieces of technology is the record that hospitals and patients maintain so that key information is accessible at all hours of the day and night.

Personal health records are becoming an important part of managing care for non-hospitalized patients as well. These secure records exist as a way to track hospital stays, outpatient appointments and medical information such as current medication lists, different medical conditions, appointments, secure messages between patients and doctors, discharge summaries, education, and health alerts or reminders. Each hospital may have a slightly different name for their own unique version of a personal health record, but during your admission the caregivers will be able to provide you with information on how to enroll, update and check your secure record after your admission.

Why does it seem like people taking care of me spend a lot of time on a computer?

With so many different types of technology in use in the hospital environment it may appear at times as if caregivers are overly interested in technology rather than interacting with their patients. The truth is that technology is constantly changing. New tools, screens and systems are frequently being introduced to help manage and communicate the ever-changing condition of patients. Caregivers are in a constant state of adapting to new features so that they can provide the best care possible.

Both hospitals and healthcare professionals are now required to ensure that they are providing high-quality care with safe patient outcomes. One of the ways in which they do this is to use a certified electronic health record (EHR). By using certified technology, caregivers and hospitals work to comply with regulatory requirements for providing care. One example of a regulatory requirement is meaningful use. Meaningful use ensures that hospitals comply with Medicare and Medicaid standards based on the ability of their caregivers to use certified electronic health records (EHR) to improve patient care. The Centers for Medicare and Medicaid Services (CMS) have established these rules because of the safety features that technology can provide. Using standardized and certified technologies ensures that alerts and notifications appear for clinicians when making critical care decisions and that consistent, high-quality care practices are used across different facilities.

What are common terms used when discussing clinical technology?

- **Medical equipment**: The hardware used in a healthcare environment to aid in the diagnosis, treatment, or monitoring of medical conditions.
- **Clinical Systems**: Computer-based systems that are designed for collecting, storing, manipulating and making available clinical information.
- **Electronic health record (EHR)**: Digital documentation of an individual's medical history and care that is maintained by health professionals and official agencies.
- **Personal health record (PHR)**: A tool that you can use to collect, track and securely share past and current information about your health or the health of someone in your care.

Are there INTERNET resources where I can learn more about health information technology?

Centers for Medicare and Medicaid Services

www.cms.gov

Health Information and Privacy (HIPAA):

http://www.hhs.gov/hipaa

Meaningful Use:

http://www.healthit.gov/providers-professionals/

meaningful-use-definition-objectives

Protected Health Information:

https://www.hipaa.com/

hipaa-protected-health-information-what-does-phi-include/

Finding Health Information via the Internet

Betsy Stovsky

L earning you have a health problem can be frightening. Maybe it's a new medical condition, or maybe you need to have a procedure. You may feel shocked, unsure of what this means for your future, how it will change your life and how it will impact you and your loved ones.

Where can I find more information?

The best source of information is your doctor, nurse or other healthcare provider. They may provide you with handouts, books, or other resources that explain the condition, treatments and what you can expect. However, it is becoming more common to use the internet to find health information. In fact, over 70% of internet users have looked online for health information at least once in the last year.

The internet is a wonderful resource for accurate health information, but it is also a source of misinformation that can cause harm when used to guide health decisions.

How do I use the internet to look for health information?

There are six points you should follow when looking for health information online.

- **Do not diagnose yourself based on what you find on the internet.** Doing so can lead to anxiety over a condition you may not have. When you have new symptoms that have been undiagnosed, start with your doctor. Do not diagnose yourself based on what you find on the internet. If you do search for symptoms, use the information to help create questions for your doctor. (See Point #6 for more information.) Just as you should not diagnose yourself, you should also avoid treating yourself without first seeing your healthcare provider.

- **Use reliable sources for information.** Look for websites that are related to national nonprofit organizations such as The American Heart Association or hospital websites (.org); government websites such as the National Library of Medicine (.gov); or an educational institution (.edu). Your doctor or hospital may have a website you can use. You can ask your doctor or nurse for words to use in your search. This also applies to sites such as YouTube, which is becoming a popular source of information. When looking at online videos, make sure they are from reputable sources.

- **Be cautious of websites that are sponsored by a product or business**. Some sponsored websites provide accurate information. For example, if you have a pacemaker and want to learn about your device, the manufacturer's website will be the best source of information about that product. However, commercial websites that are selling a product may be biased toward the product and make claims that are exaggerated or out of context. Be cautious and check the sources for credibility.

- **Use current information.** There should be a date listed on the web page. Health information changes daily, so it is important to make sure you access the most up-to-date information. Research may reveal that some treatments or ways to manage health conditions, even those that have been in practice for years, are now outdated or even harmful.

- **Look for the Health on the Net Foundation Code of Conduct (HONcode).** This is the stamp of approval for medical and health websites. It ensures that the website is following eight principles of credible and reliable health information.
- **Use your information as if you were a detective or a reporter.** Keep your information in a folder along with your medical history and medication list. Use the information to make a list of questions to take to your doctor's appointment. Helpful questions are:

  - Is this my diagnosis?
  - Will I need any tests to confirm my diagnosis?
  - What treatment options listed apply to me? What are my specific risks and benefits for each option? How successful are the treatments?
  - How will this diagnosis change my lifestyle? Are there changes I need to make?

The Agency for Healthcare Quality and Research *http://www.ahrq. gov/patients-consumers/patient-involvement/ask-your-doctor/questions-during-appointment.html* offers sample questions you can ask so that you have a good understanding of what you need to know in order to follow the doctor's recommendations.

What kinds of support groups are available?

You may find it helpful to join an online support group. Talking to others who share your experience can help you understand what your condition means to you as a person and what to expect from treatments and procedures. Support groups are particularly helpful for patients with rare disorders. They can keep you informed about the latest research and treatments and be a source of information when little else is available. But, keep these tips in mind:

- **Read some of the questions and answers before you participate.** Make sure the responses are helpful and supportive, not angry or mean-spirited. If the support group has been around for some time, it is nice to know people felt comfortable enough to stick around and help others.
- **Protect your privacy**. You may be required to sign on to the site. Choose a user name that does not provide links to your personal information. Do not provide personal information about where you live, your email address or phone number.
- **Remember that the point of the site is to provide support**. Not all people have the same medical history or react to treatments in the same way. Do not take medical advice from others, such as "**Don't** take that medication; I had a terrible reaction to it." or "**Take** a pill or supplement; it saved my life." Do not start or stop any treatment without first talking to your doctor or the caregiver that prescribed it.
- Remember that everyone's illness experience is different. Just because someone else had a bad outcome does not mean that you will, too.

Ask your doctor, nurse or social worker if they can recommend reliable, helpful support groups.

How do I choose the best place to have a treatment or procedure?

Research shows that when having surgery, you should choose a location where there are many procedures performed similar to the one you need. In addition to a high volume of procedures, you should look for a location that has multidisciplinary practices. It is likely that you have more than one medical condition and need an experienced team of doctors and nurses who can address all your healthcare needs when you have surgery. The first step is to ask your doctor for a recommendation. If you want to "shop" online, here are some things to look for:

- **Search for information on volume, experience and success rates of the hospital and surgeon.** These are called outcomes. Many hospitals publish outcomes online. Common ways to measure success are:
  - ✓ **Mortality.** This is the death rate related to a procedure.
  - ✓ **Morbidity.** This is a measurement of how many patients had complications related to a procedure.

- Search for information about the department and surgeon, as well as patient satisfaction.
- Look for information related to hospital ratings from:
  - ✓ **Joint Commission** - http://www.jointcommission.org/
  - ✓ **Medicare** - http://medicare.gov/hospitalcompare/search.html
  - ✓ **National organizations.** Many national professional organizations have listings of hospitals, benchmarks, and methods to assess patient safety. For example, the Society of Thoracic Surgeons looks at quality and patient safety related to heart procedures. This information is published on their website, http://www.sts.org/quality-research-patient-safety

Can I trust health information I get from TV shows and the news?

Don't believe **everything** you see and hear! Take notes. Bring your notes to your next appointment and discuss what you found with the doctor or nurse. Not all studies are created equal. Find out how many people were included in the study. Was the report based on information from a randomized controlled study (the gold standard of research), an observational study (by chance), or an analysis of multiple studies (meta-analysis)? Randomized controlled studies use specific research questions and controlled conditions to learn more about a treatment or condition (answer a research question). The other two types of studies are great ways to discover a trend for future research, but they may not provide answers to the specific research question. Find out if the research was published in a top peer-reviewed journal, which is a sign that it is a more highly regarded study.

As mentioned before, new studies are published every day. New research leads to more information about conditions and possible treatments. But, again, it is important not to ever change your medication or treatment plan without first talking to your doctor.

What other resources can I use to learn more?

In addition to your doctor's office and online resources, you may find these resources helpful:

- **Online Health Chats**. Online health chats give you the opportunity to ask a healthcare professional specific questions. They are scheduled several times a month and may be text-based or video-based.
- **A nurse or health educator**. Some hospital websites and insurance companies offer the opportunity to ask a nurse or health educator questions in a private setting— either by phone or online through live-chat technology.

It is important for you and your family to be involved in your healthcare. There is even a term for this — the e-patient — one who is educated, empowered and engaged in their healthcare. The goal of being an e-patient is to participate in your healthcare so you can have the best possible outcomes. Making sure you have all the information tools in your patient toolkit is one of the first steps to becoming a full partner in your care.

Are there INTERNET resources where I can learn more about patient education resources?

MedlinePlus (National Library of Medicine) -
https://www.nia.nih.gov/health

National Institute of Health -
https://www.nih.gov/health-information

Healthfinder.gov -
https://healthfinder.gov/

Center for Disease Control and Prevention -
https://www.cdc.gov/

National Institute on Aging -
https://www.nia.nih.gov/health

American Academy of Pediatrics -
https://www.healthychildren.org/English/Pages/default.aspx

National organizations such as:

- American Diabetes Association
  http://www.diabetes.org/

- American Heart Association
  http://www.heart.org/HEARTORG/

- American Cancer Society
  https://www.cancer.org//

Preparing Your Children or Grandchildren for Your Hospitalization

Meredith Lahl

Young children and grandchildren have many questions when their parent or grandparent is in the hospital. A hospitalized parent or grandparent interrupts the daily routine and can cause the child to become fearful and worried. It is important to share as much information as possible according to their age. How children react to an ill or hospitalized parent varies greatly with their age. They ultimately want to know how the illness relates to them. This is a normal developmental thought process.

What are some considerations in beginning a conversation with my child or grandchild?

- The child's age
- The severity and nature of the illness
- Whether this was a sudden episode or planned hospitalization
- How long you will be away from your child
- How your child's daily routine will be affected by the hospitalization

- Who will provide the care or support that you generally provide to the child
- The type of hospital environment in which you will be receiving care – intensive care, non-intensive care, post-partum, hospice, etc.

What important guidelines should I use when talking with my children/grandchildren?

First and foremost, always be honest. If you choose to minimize details the child may become fearful of information you will share in the future. Offer information in small amounts, and do not hide information. Children often overhear an adult's conversation and make scary assumptions on their own.

Children may ask direct questions such as "Are you going to die?" or "Do you have cancer?" Answer all questions as best as you can but don't give more of an answer to the question than what was asked. It is okay to say that you do not know.

Although it is natural to want to provide hopeful information, avoid making promises that you may not be able to keep. Do not assure a child that you will be present for an important event if you are not sure you will be out of the hospital or strong enough to do so. This could damage the child's trust in you. If you must answer this type of question, tell the child that you will do your best.

Ask the hospital if there is an opportunity for the child to see an empty room or other equipment that is not being used by a patient. Many hospitals have resources such as child life specialists to help prepare children for what they will see when they visit.

There are many books available to help younger children understand a parent's or grandparent's illness.

What might my children/grandchildren be thinking about?

- Are you going to die?
- Will you be able to take care of me?
- Who will take care of me?
- Did I cause this to happen?
- Who is going to feed me?
- Who is going to pick me up from school?
- Who is going to wash my clothes?
- Who is going to put my hair in a ponytail in the morning before school?

How should I expect my children/grandchildren to react?

Each child will react differently based on many factors. Their relationship with you also determines their reaction. If you are their primary caretaker, there will be much concern for what will happen to them. Some children will become withdrawn, while others may act out or become aggressive at home or school. You will want to consider all behaviors and be aware of direct and indirect responses.

What are some things I can do to help my child cope?

- Maintain a sense of normalcy with routines, caretakers and activities. This has been identified as the most helpful coping strategy for children.
- Maintain established limits in the home. Children respond to limits best.
- Help your children and grandchildren understand that it is OK to continue to play with friends and enjoy activities that they enjoyed before you were hospitalized. They may feel guilty for doing so.
- If you are in the hospital for an extended period of time, allow children to visit on their terms while recognizing how you are feeling.

- When children do visit, spend protected time with them doing things you would do at home with them, such as making puzzles, coloring, listening to music or watching a favorite TV show.
- Your child or grandchild may not know how to act around your or help you. Be as patient as possible and guide them so that they feel valued and important.
- Take advantage of technology and arrange for frequent visits via video calling.

How do I know if they need more help managing?

Children will show signs of stress or worry by changing their eating or sleeping patterns, having night terrors or tantrums or becoming quieter. Children may also regress. For example, a child who has been toilet trained will begin to wet their pants or bed.

What can I expect when I go home?

- Your child will have possibly met certain milestones, met certain goals or had accomplishments at school or their activities that you missed. It is important to be proud of those milestones and goals and to support children.
- Begin to work with other caregivers in the home to re-establish a routine. Your children and grandchildren may have gotten used to a different caregiver and will need time to re-adjust.
- Children may reject you or punish you for being away. Although this can feel hurtful it is developmentally appropriate. Do not take this personally.

Are there internet resources where I can learn more about helping children cope with a parent or grandparent's hospitalization?

The Child Life Council
https://www.childlife.org/

The American Academy of Pediatrics
www.aap.org

Part Two:

Identifying Nursing Care Practices: Comfort, Safety and Education

"The nurse is temporarily the consciousness of the unconscious, the love of life for the suicidal, the leg of the amputee, the eyes of the newly blind, a means of locomotion for the infant, the knowledge and confidence of the young mother, and a voice for those too weak to speak."

Virginia Henderson, RN

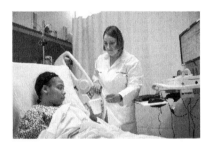
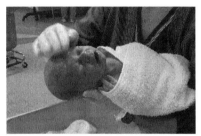
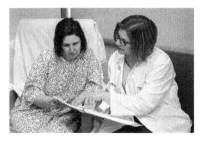
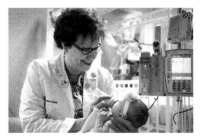

Protecting Against Infection

Monica Weber

Prevention of infection while hospitalized is a fundamental activity for all healthcare providers. Since the 1800s, handwashing has been the cornerstone of infection protection. However, with the increasing use of technology and equipment, it has become evident that excellent handwashing by all caregivers is not enough to prevent infection.

What impact does the hospital environment have on my risk of infection?

Handwashing (also known as hand hygiene) reduces the number of bacteria on the hands. While much of infection prevention has focused on caregivers washing their hands in between touching patients, it is equally important for patients and their visitors to keep their hands clean. Your nurse should offer you an opportunity to wash your hands before and after eating or using the bathroom. Handwashing does not eliminate all germs from the skin but instead reduces the number so that anyone touching equipment or the environment will not add to the amount of germs that are already present. In addition to hand hygiene, the hospital environment is another area that caregivers and hospital executives monitor in order to prevent infections and the spread of infections in the hospital.

The hospital environment is not sterile, but your caregivers will carefully clean the environment and equipment around you to reduce exposure to germs. Housekeeping or environmental services will clean your hospital room daily, focusing on the bathroom and areas that you touch frequently, such as the phone or your bed controls. They utilize cleaning products that are made to reduce germs in the hospital environment. Some types of infections require the environmental service workers to utilize bleach solution to fight particularly resistant germs, such as clostrium difficile (C-diff). Nursing staff are responsible for cleaning the equipment that touches your skin in between patients. You may see them utilize medicated wipes, similar to baby wipes, to clean equipment such as thermometers and blood pressure cuffs in between patient use.

What is considered good hand hygiene?

Hand hygiene is either done by washing hands for 15-20 seconds with soap and water or using alcohol-based hand rubs. Alternative products are available, but all of the guidelines for healthcare recommend alcohol-based products. With few exceptions, either handwashing or the use of hand rubs is acceptable. The exceptions include before or after using the restroom, handling bodily fluids, or certain kinds of infection such as C-diff. Soap in the hospital is antibacterial, but antibacterial soap or other products are not necessary in the home environment. The action of rubbing is more important for removal of germs than the small amount of antibacterial product in soap products.

Hands should be wet with water before applying soap, then all surfaces are lathered and rinsed with the water flowing downward off of the hands. Hands are dried, being careful to not recontaminate the hands when turning off the faucet. With hand rubs, it is important to use enough product to cover all surfaces of the hands, particularly in between the fingers and around the nail beds. The product should be rubbed in until it is dry.

Hospitals monitor hand hygiene frequency in a variety of ways. They may do random observations or utilize technology to count and remind caregivers to wash their hands when entering or exiting the patient's room. It is perfectly acceptable to ask a caregiver if they have washed their hands before they touch you, although patients may feel reluctant to do so. All caregivers are aware of the importance of handwashing, but in the busy care environment may simply forget. The response to the question about hand hygiene should be "thank you."

What about personal protective equipment and precautions?

Gloves are used to protect caregivers from exposure to infectious bodily fluids as well as reduce contamination of the hands. You should expect everyone to clean their hands before putting on gloves as well as after taking gloves off. Gloves should be changed when going from a dirty to a clean area of the body. It is generally not necessary for visitors to wear gloves unless they are performing physical care for the patient or if the patient is in isolation for an infectious disease.

If a patient is hospitalized or develops certain infections, he or she may be placed into physical precautions (formerly called isolation). Precautions are based on the type and site of the infection. For instance, tuberculosis may be spread through the air, so patients are kept in a private room with special air exchange. Anyone entering the room will be asked to wear a mask. On the other hand, if a patient develops C-diff (clostrium difficile, which may cause an infection of the lining of the colon), everyone entering the room will be asked to wear a gown and gloves and wash their hands only with soap and water, not a hand rub. Signs are placed on the door to the patient room, and nursing staff will instruct patients and families as to what precautions (gown, gloves, masks) are necessary.

When in precautions it is vital for the patient and visitors to follow the specific precautions carefully to prevent exposure to themselves and prevent the spread of infection to other patients or hospital staff. Patients in precautions may feel isolated because the door to their room must be kept closed and also because they may only see caregivers and visitors through gowns and gloves. Nurses and infection prevention specialists will monitor the laboratory tests and condition of the patient to determine when the patient may be removed from the precautions.

What are other fundamental principles of infection prevention?

The skin is a protective organ that serves as a vital barrier against infection. Once the integrity of the skin has been broken by a surgical incision or an intravenous (IV) line, bacteria and viruses may enter the blood and cause an infection. Therefore, great care is taken to clean the skin prior to surgery and to keep surgical incisions clean, dry and covered until initial healing has taken place, typically within 1-2 days.

Recent studies have shown that patients in intensive care units who have many IV lines and tubes in their bodies will have fewer infections if they are bathed with a certain type of soap that is used to cleanse the skin prior to surgery. These patients may also have the inside of their noses swabbed to check for bacteria that may also predispose them to acquiring infections after surgery or in the ICU.

The key point is that nurses and doctors will thoughtfully evaluate whether the patient needs an IV line before it is inserted and also make every attempt to remove any IV or tubes as soon as they are no longer necessary.

What is done to protect me from an infection if I need a line or tube?

If a line or tube is necessary, several actions will reduce the chance of an infection. During insertion of IV lines into large veins (also known as a central line), doctors and nurses will wear surgical gowns, masks and gloves during the procedure. If you are awake they may ask you to wear a mask over your nose and mouth as well or at least to turn your head away from the site. Skin is cleaned with the same kind of soap as during surgery. Once the IV line is inserted they will apply a dressing (bandage) over the site to keep it clean and dry and to keep the skin free of germs. Before an IV line is used to give a medication, nurses will vigorously clean the line with alcohol to prevent germs from entering the line.

Tubes such as urinary catheters to drain urine (known as foley catheters) are removed as soon as possible to reduce the risk of a urinary tract infection. Even a few years ago a urinary catheter would be kept in place to make it easier on the patient to go to the bathroom while bedridden, but now the tubes are removed as soon as possible to prevent infection. During insertion, the area is cleansed and the tube is secured. There are some occasions where a urinary catheter needs to be kept in place because of certain surgeries or conditions, such as a bladder that is unable to fully empty your urine. In this case, to prevent infection the nursing staff will keep the drainage bag hanging down so no urine flows back into the bladder, but not so low as to touch the floor. Every day the area around the catheter should be cleaned. If you need to go home with it, the nurse should give you instructions on how to prevent and recognize infection.

What will happen if I do develop an infection?

Patients are usually in the hospital so that they can be monitored as they recover from an illness or surgery. The nursing staff will monitor your heart rate, blood pressure, respirations and temperature as a way to identify early signs of an infection. Laboratory studies such as white blood count are also monitored. All incisions and insertion sites of any tubes or IV are carefully inspected during dressing changes to identify early signs of infection. Antibiotics are given to prevent infection immediately after surgery, but are no longer given more than a day or two after surgery. Should there be a suspicion of an infection, your nurses and doctors will monitor your vital signs more frequently and may administer antibiotics that treat the most likely type of bacteria until the actual bacteria is known.

Besides an IV line infection (central line infection) or urinary catheter infection (urinary tract infection), patients who undergo surgical procedures or must remain in bed for extended periods of time are at risk of developing pneumonia. Pneumonia is an infection of the lungs. Prevention of pneumonia is a partnership between the patient and the caregiving team. All patients benefit by getting up and moving as soon as possible. Movement stimulates deep breathing which opens up the lung sacs and prevents accumulation of mucus. Movement also drops the diaphragm allowing for deeper breaths. Patients in the intensive care unit with a breathing tube will also have the head of their beds elevated up to at least 30 degrees to mimic the effect of movement.

Another action to prevent pneumonia is good oral hygiene. If you have a breathing tube, nurses will clean your mouth every hour with the tube in place and suction your lungs. If you don't have a breathing tube, teeth and gums will be cleaned normally. Recent studies have begun to link gingivitis (red and swollen gums) to conditions other than just infection such as heart disease, uncontrolled diabetes or premature birth. A visit to dentist is not only good for your smile, but it improves overall health.

What can I do to prevent infections when I'm not in the hospital?

Your mother was right; staying healthy is the best defense against infection. Your immune system is highly effective against exposure to germs, so eating right, exercising and common sense go far to protect you. Modern science has given the medical field additional tools with which to prevent and treat infections.

Vaccines are an important part of prevention. You should make sure that you receive a flu shot every year and a pneumonia vaccine if you are over the age of 65 or have a chronic medical condition. Obtain the suggested vaccines for your children to protect them and you as well.

If you do develop an infection, ask the doctor if an antibiotic is necessary and if so, take it exactly as prescribed. Do not stop when you start to feel better because if you relapse, you risk requiring a much longer course of treatment in the future. The converse is true as well. Do not insist upon antibiotics unless they are indicated for your conditions. For instance, colds and the flu are caused by viruses, and antibiotics do not work against viruses. In addition, needless antibiotics are a significant cause of antibiotic resistance. Certain bacteria have mutated, so the usual antibiotics are no longer effective without the prospect of many new antibiotics in development.

If you are the visitor and not the patient, please stay away if you are sick. Patients in the hospital are at increased risk for additional infections. Wearing a mask if you have a cold may make sense if you must see the patient but is not perfect protection.

The final word is to partner with your caregiving team. Understand your specific risk, especially if you have a chronic medical condition. If you are healthy, work with your nurses and doctors to stay that way.

Before going home, you should be able to answer "YES" to all of the following statements:

> ✓ I know the importance of washing my hands
> ✓ I know the importance of keeping up with immunizations
> ✓ I know the difference between a viral and bacterial infection

What INTERNET resources are available where I can learn more about handwashing practices in the hospital?

Centers for Disease Control and Prevention – hand hygiene
www.cdc.gov/handhygiene

Joint Commission - hand hygiene SPEAKUP Program
www.jointcommission.org/topics/hai_hand_hygeine.aspx

World Health Organization/
http://www.who.int/gpsc/tools/faqs/evidence_hand_hygiene/en/

Administering Medications Safely

Catherine Skowronsky, Jennifer Colwill & Christian Burchill

During your stay you will likely receive medications intended to help you manage your illness. In this chapter, you will learn what to expect during your hospitalization regarding taking medications and learning their purpose. An uneventful hospital stay actually begins before admission.

Here are four things to help you prepare for your admission regarding medication safety:

- Bring a list of current medications with you. The list should include the names, doses, routes (the way a medication is taken, such as by mouth/orally) and frequency of all of your prescription medications as well as over-the-counter and herbal supplements.
- Make a list if you don't have one. Bring more than one copy that you can share with your caregivers.
- Keep this list accessible to family and Emergency Medical Services (EMS) in case of an emergency. Place it near the entryway of your home, on the refrigerator or in your spouses' purse or wallet, for example.

- Enlist the help of a care partner. This can be a spouse, friend, neighbor or relative. This is someone you trust to speak on your behalf, who can share your medication routine in case you would become too ill to speak for yourself.

What does your nurse need to know about you?

As mentioned in an earlier chapter, when you are admitted to the hospital you will be asked a lot of questions by many individuals. Many of the questions are about the medications you take at home. Be ready to share the names, doses, frequency of all of your medications and any allergies you may have to certain medications. This includes herbals, homeopathic/natural remedies and over the counter treatments. Please tell your caregivers if you have stopped taking any of your medications. If financial complications have prevented you from taking your medications as prescribed, please share this information. Medications can only help you if you can afford to take them. When it comes to your medications, open and honest communication is best.

How will my medications be managed while I am in the hospital?

Your physician, nurse practitioner or physician's assistant will review the medications you take at home and determine whether or not these medications and dosages will be continued in the hospital based upon your physical condition.

The nurse is responsible for reviewing and safely administering your medications as prescribed by the doctor. If the nurse has any concerns regarding what is prescribed, he or she will have a conversation with your doctor and recommend any changes to keep you safe. Here is what you should expect each time you receive medication in the hospital:

Your bedside nurse will:

- Verify your name and date of birth.
- Review your allergies against the medications to keep you safe.
- Tell you the name and dose of every medication.
- Teach you about the purpose of every medication and possible side effects.

The pharmacist reviews every medication ordered for you. He or she looks for harmful interactions and compares the prescriptions with your allergies to keep you safe. The pharmacist can also teach you about the medications you are taking. Throughout your hospital stay, the types of medications and doses may change depending on your response to them.

What can I do to prevent a medication error?

Know the medications you are being given while in the hospital. If you are too sick, your loved ones should know this information. Ask the nurse before you take the medication what each drug is for and why you are taking it. The nurse will verify your name and date of birth before giving you any medication. Some hospitals have special equipment that scans the drug and your patient ID band to ensure that the right patient is getting the correct medications at the right time.

How do I know if my medication is working?

Your bedside nurse will monitor you for signs that the medications are working as intended without harmful side effects. This monitoring may include checking your blood pressure more frequently than at home, keeping track of how much urine you are making in a day, observing how steady you are as you walk down the hall and noticing a change in your appetite. Since your nurse spends more time with you than other members of your healthcare team, he or she will be collecting important pieces of information that will identify your progress. Your nurse will share this information with other caregivers so that everyone is well informed of your condition. Sometimes patients do not want to "bother" the nurse by sharing something that may seem trivial. However, any change or worry about your health should be shared so that your concerns can be explored.

How will I learn about my medications?

You can expect every one of your bedside nurses to discuss your medications with you in order to determine whether you have the correct information to take your medications safely. This may seem repetitive, but it is important that you have a good understanding of your medications. Here are some of the main pieces of information you can expect to hear.

- What is the reason for taking a particular medication?
- What are some of the main possible side effects associated with a medication?
- What to do if there is a problem with your medications?

Some medications require learning special skills such as giving yourself an injection, using an inhaler, applying a medicated patch or receiving your medications via a feeding tube. Ask early in your stay when you or your loved one is going to learn these skills. Your nurse or pharmacist will teach you the proper skills while you are in the hospital. This should not be a one-time lesson. After the instruction, you or your loved one should perform this skill so you have confidence to do it at home.

What should I do if I do not plan to take a medication that has been prescribed for me?

If at any time, you know of a reason why you would not take a medication as prescribed, please say so. An honest patient is his or her own best advocate. You may have cultural or other personal reasons for the decision that a particular drug is not right for you. Your caregiving team will work with you to find an alternative therapy whenever possible. If you have concerns about paying for your medications, a social worker or case manager can help find resources. Research has shown that a third of patients never get their prescriptions filled.

What do I need to know before I go home?

Good news. You're discharged from the hospital. That means that you can sleep in your own bed, eat your own food and take your own medications. An important part of the discharge process is when your nurse reviews your medications with you and your loved ones. Many of the medications you will be taking at home are not new to you. This is a good time to ask your caregivers about what to do with your old medications. This may be especially true if you are taking the same medication but a different dose. Avoid breaking, crushing or chewing tablets without asking your pharmacist, doctor or nurse. It may be possible for the hospital to fill any new prescriptions before you leave.

How can I be successful in taking my medications at home?

Before going home, you should be able to answer "YES" to all of the following statements:

✓ I know the names, dosages, side effects and directions for taking ALL my medications that have been prescribed.

✓ I know how to prepare this medication in order to take it correctly – crush, dissolve, mix, dilute, etc.

✓ I know why this (these) medication(s) were prescribed for me.

✓ I know what actions to take if I miss a dose of my medication.

✓ I know how to get this medication refilled.

✓ I know how long I need to take this medication.

✓ I know what to do with my old medications at home.

✓ I know the restrictions to follow when taking these medications (such as diet, exercise, bleeding risk, intimacy, driving, or operating heavy equipment).

✓ I know how I am going to pay for this medication.

✓ I know how to properly store this medication at home so that it is not damaged.

✓ I know which foods affect the way my medication works.

✓ I know how alcohol affects the way my medication works.

✓ I know not to take any more or less than the prescribed dose.

✓ I know what side effects to watch out for.

✓ I know when and whom to call if I am having a major side effect from my medication.

✓ I know who is going to help me take my medications at home if I need assistance.

✓ I know how to use the equipment that is needed to administer my medication – inhalers, syringes, patches, pumps, etc.

✓ I have an established routine to take my medications as prescribed.

✓ I know how to get y prescription(s) refilled

You're home. Now what?

So now you are home! Here are some important things you can do so you have the best chance of staying home, the best place to be!

1. **Get organized**. Keep all of the notes and discharge information that you received from the hospital in a safe place that you can easily find. Take out the list of medications and important numbers to call and put them in a place where you can easily see them. The refrigerator is a common place.

   Remember to fill your prescriptions if you have not already. You cannot take your medications if you do not have them!

   Develop a plan to take the next dose if you take a medication more than once a day. Enlist the help of your loved ones to come up with a plan. Schedule your medications around your daily activities. Make a list or use a reminder application on your phone. Find a strategy that works for you.

2. **Store your mediations as directed**. Keep all of your medications close to one another or where you plan to be when you take them. For example, if one medication is refrigerated, keep the others nearby if you plan to take them together. Medications ordered at bed time or first thing in the morning can be placed on the nightstand or dresser if you do not have small children. Avoid keeping them in the bathroom. The humid environment can impair how well the medication works. Discuss with your pharmacist where and how the medications should be stored.

   Purchase and use a pill sorter. Pill sorters come in a variety of sizes and hold anywhere from a day's worth of medication to all the medication you take in a month.

3. **Keep your medication list up to date**. Revise your medication list with any new medications or dose changes you brought home from the hospital. Make sure to bring it along to all of your follow-up appointments. If you see more than one doctor, take it to each one so that all of your doctors can update their own records. Always ask if your doctor wants you to make any changes to your medications before leaving your appointment.

How can I be successful in taking my medications?

Taking medications as prescribed is an important activity in keeping you well or helping you recover. Your doctor has determined that you need this medication to prevent complications or control the symptoms of your condition. Do not take more medication than prescribed as the dose has been determined based upon your age, weight and condition. More is not better. Follow the directions on your medication. If you do not understand, ask the pharmacist before you pay for your medication. Pharmacy staff now ask if you have any questions for the pharmacist. You must answer yes or no in order to purchase your medications.

There may be times when you just don't want to take your medications. If you are experiencing these feelings and as a result not taking your medications as prescribed, you need to discuss this with your physician or healthcare provider. Any decision to change or stop medications should be in collaboration with a healthcare provider who knows your condition and your overall health status. Medication management of any illness is crucial to your long-term health.

Taking your medications correctly is one of the most important things you can do to stay healthy and manage the symptoms of your disease. Learning about your medications is an ongoing process. It is important to keep learning more about your condition and things that you can do to maintain your health. It is also important to keep learning about your medications and how they help you manage your illness. Understanding them helps you and your caregiving team manage medications instead of the medications managing your life.

Are there INTERNET resources where I can learn more about medication safety?

Centers for Disease Control and Prevention Medication Safety Program
http://www.cdc.gov/medicationsafety/

Food and Drug Administration, Information for Consumers
http://www.fda.gov/Drugs/ResourcesForYou/Consumers/default.htm

Institute for Safe Medication Practices
http://www.ismp.org/tools/

Managing Pain

Sandra Siedlecki

There are different types of pain (acute or chronic) and any number of problems that can cause pain. For example, patients can have pain due to a disease process (diabetes or infection), an injury (fractures or lacerations) or a surgical or interventional procedure. Regardless of the cause, patients have the right to expect their caregivers will work with them to manage their pain. Because of recent advances in healthcare, most patients today can receive an acceptable level of pain relief.

What is an acceptable level of pain relief?

While it would be wonderful to be able to eliminate pain for all patients during their entire stay, that is not always possible. We are limited in part by the side effects of pain medications. They can make patients excessively sleepy, affect the respiratory muscles and compromise breathing. However, it is not unreasonable to expect your pain to be managed at a level that allows you to be somewhat comfortable, even if you are not totally pain free.

How will my pain be assessed?

Pain is a very subjective experience, and the patient is the expert. Only the patient can determine how much pain they are having, where it is located and how it feels. Whenever possible the pain assessment is based upon the patient's self-report. Besides describing your pain, the nurse or doctor should ask you about pain medications you have had in the past and how well they worked, any problems you experienced (side effects) or other information that will help them select the best treatment plan for you.

Pain is assessed in several ways. The nurse or doctor may ask you first to point to the location of the pain and tell them if the pain is sharp, dull, radiating, non-radiating, burning, aching, or some other adjective. It is important to describe your pain carefully because it can help your health-care provider assess the possible cause(s) of the pain and direct them in selecting the best method to manage your pain.

In addition to assessing the location and quality of your pain, your nurse or doctor will ask you to rate your pain on a scale from zero (0) to ten (10), with zero indicating no pain and ten indicating the worst pain you could imagine. This verbal pain scale can be repeated frequently to gauge how well your pain is being controlled.

How will my pain be reassessed?

Ideally, we would like to manage your pain at a level of three (3) or less. But the side effects of pain medication may not make this possible. During one of your initial pain assessments, the doctor or nurse will ask you your expectations about pain management during your hospitalization. They will ask you to tell them on a scale from zero (0) to ten (10) what number represents an acceptable level of pain management to you. It is OK to be honest with the doctor or nurse when you are asked this question.

What if my pain exceeds the verbal rating scale choices?

While it is not usual, some patients have pain that they rate way beyond the zero (0) to ten (10) scale. If this occurs, it is OK to tell the doctor and nurse that your pain is beyond the worst pain you could have imagined (10). You may in this case rate your pain at a level above the scale (11, 12, or higher). The reason we want to know this information is so we can later assess if our treatment has resulted in any improvement. A decrease in pain from 12 to 10 is important, but doctors and nurses can only know this if we know what level your pain was at before the treatment.

What if the patient cannot speak?

Although self-report is the best way to assess pain, doctors and nurses have at their disposal other resources to assess pain in patients who are not able to verbalize their pain. Several assessment tools have been developed and are used to estimate pain for these patients. Another way to estimate pain for non-verbal patients is to consider their circumstances and provide pain medication appropriately. For example, patients who have surgery experience pain, so it would be expected that even if you cannot speak and tell us about your pain, you are still experiencing pain after your surgery.

What if the patient is confused?

Although assessing pain for individuals who are confused can be a challenge, there are ways to estimate and assess pain in these individuals. Research has shown that even confused patients can be asked if they have pain. Although they may not be capable of describing it or providing a number to describe the quantity of pain, they can usually provide a location. Other indications can be a general change in behavior: for example, sedate patients become agitated, and agitated patients become sedate.

What if I have chronic pain?

Patients who have an underlying chronic pain condition controlled at home with a specific medication regimen should share this information with doctor and nurses. Ideally chronic pain medications should be continued during hospitalization. However, circumstances may impact your caregiver's ability to do this. For example, if the medication is not something the hospital stores in its pharmacy, doctors might change the medication to a similar medication; or they may ask your family to bring in your prescription so they can lock it up and administer it during your hospitalization.

> **IMPORTANT NOTE:** It is critical that you do not self-medicate while you are a patient in the hospital, as there may be potential undesired actions with other medication that you are not aware of.

Should you ask your doctor and nurses questions about your pain and your pain management treatment plan?

You are a partner in your care. To be a full partner, you need to ask your doctor and nurse questions about your pain management treatment plan. Some things you might ask include:

- How long should I expect the pain to last?
- What things should I report immediately?
- What pain medications have been prescribed?
- How often will I be given or at least offered my pain medication?
- Do I have to ask for my pain medication, or will the nurse just bring it in when it is time?
- If the routine pain medication is not helping can I have additional medications in between pain medication doses?

What types of pain medication might be ordered?

Pain medications fall into several classes and can be given orally, as an injection (rarely) or intravenously. The route selected by your healthcare provider will be based in part on you and your condition. For example, sometimes patients are not allowed to eat nor have fluids (called NPO). For patients who cannot take food or fluids or for whom food and fluids are not currently recommended, we can administer the medication into a muscle (injection) or a vein (intravenous). Some medications come in only one form (oral or intravenous only), so availability will also impact treatment decisions.

Opioids: The most potent type of pain medication is often referred to as an opioid. Laypeople might call these narcotics, although that is not really the correct terminology. Opioids are used to treat moderate to severe pain.

- **Routes of Administration**: While these pain medications are often available for both oral and intravenous administration, they are typically given intravenously initially. Once pain is controlled, the treatment plan may indicate that the pain medication can be switched from intravenous to oral. Ideally, managing pain with oral medications is the treatment of choice.
- **Side Effects**: Opioid medication has side effects, and their use is often limited by these side effects. The nurse will monitor you for these side effects, which may include:

  - **Nausea** (with or without vomiting): Some opioids cause more nausea than others. If this becomes a problem, let your nurse or doctor know so they can either adjust your dose or change to a different opioid.
  - **Constipation**: Most pain medications result in some constipation, so patients prescribed opioids are often also prescribed a stool softener. If you are not receiving a stool softener or if the stool softener is not working and you believe you are

constipated or becoming constipated, please let your doctor or nurse know.

- ○ **Respiratory depression and excessive sedation**: The dose and frequency with which we can administer opioid medication for pain is primarily limited by your response to the medication side effects. Respiratory depression and excessive sedation is not necessarily dose related; some people can experience respiratory depression and excessive sedation the very first time they receive an opioid medication, regardless of dose. Each individual is very different, and size does not seem to be associated with how well you do or do not tolerate opioid medications. Because of this, the nurse will closely monitor your sedation level after administering an opioid medication.

How does the nurse assess my sedation level?

Because research suggests that excessive sedation comes before respiratory depression (which is very serious), nurses routinely monitor a patient who has received any opioid medications. To perform this assessment, the nurse observes the patient and rates the observations on a scale from 0 to -5. A zero rating means the patient is alert and calm. If the patient is drowsy, but has sustained periods of being awake and is able to open their eyes in response to a verbal command by the nurse, their sedation level is rated -1. Light sedation (-2) is assessed as a patient who wakes easily but briefly while opening their eyes in response to a verbal command by the nurse.

These first three levels are typically seen in a patient who is being treated with opioid medications and is normal. The last two levels of sedation – deep sedation and unarousable – are not normal responses and require action on the part of the nurse and doctor. Patients whose sedation level is -4 or -5 would not be given any opioid medication until their sedation level improved and may require administration of a drug called Narcan to decrease the effect of the opioid and decrease the sedation level. If you notice excessive sedation in your family member who has received an opioid medication, you should always notify your nurse right away.

What other medications are given for pain?

Mild to moderate pain is typically treated with oral medications that contain some opioid medications but at lower doses than the medications given for moderate to severe pain. These medications are thought to act by decreasing inflammation. You may know them by their more common names: Tylenol® (Acetaminophen) and Motrin® (Ibuprofen). It is important to remember that just because these medications are available over-the-counter, they are still potentially dangerous. For example, Tylenol® is metabolized by your liver; too much Tylenol® can damage your liver and actually cause liver failure.

It is recommended that you not take more than 4,000 mg of Tylenol® per day (one extra-strength Tylenol® has 1,000 mg) and not take Tylenol® routinely for prolonged periods of time. Motrin® has similar potential problems related to dose and duration of use. In addition to Tylenol® and Motrin®, your healthcare provider may order other medications, such as antidepressants, in low doses or anti-anxiety medications that have been found to be useful for certain types of pain.

Is there anything else I can do for the pain, other than taking medications?

There are many complementary treatments you can use to help manage your pain while in the hospital. Below are just a few:

- Change your position every 1 to 2 hours, and get up and moving as soon as possible after procedures and surgery.
- Ask the nurse to help position you with additional pillows for comfort; the position of comfort will be related to the cause of your pain.

- Ask your family to bring in music and headsets so you can use this to help manage your pain. There is significant research to support the use of music for pain control. You can select music that makes you feel a certain way. So if you feel tight and tense, listen to music that makes you feel relaxed. If you lack energy and feel sluggish all of the time, listen to music that makes you feel energized. If you cannot sleep, listen to music that is restful. If you are sad or depressed, listen to music that is uplifting. Preferences for music are unique, and what one person perceives as music may be noise to someone else. Listen to music that speaks to you. But listen with headsets so you do not bother others.

- Watch TV, read and talk with friends in person or on the phone. These may be useful distraction techniques to manage mild to moderate pain.

- Use breathing exercises or relaxation techniques to help you rest and decrease pain. Deep breathing relaxation techniques include the following:

  ✓ Sit comfortably with your back straight. Put one hand on your chest and the other on your stomach.

  ✓ Breathe in through your nose. The hand on your stomach should rise. The hand on your chest should move very little.

  ✓ Exhale through your mouth, pushing out as much air as you can while contracting your abdominal muscles. The hand on your stomach should move in as you exhale, but your other hand should move very little.

  ✓ Continue to breathe in through your nose and out through your mouth. Try to inhale enough so that your lower abdomen rises and falls. Count slowly as you exhale.

- Massage (hand, foot or body), guided imagery and Reiki or therapeutic touch require assistance from someone trained in these procedures. However, many people find that they help them to manage their pain. Many hospitals are now beginning to provide access to these services to patients. To find out if your hospital has these services, ask your nurse.

Remember, pain can be managed. You should be an active participant in your care by asking questions and providing important information to your caregivers. Nurses care about your experiences and outcomes, and they are there to help. Just ask.

How can I manage my pain at home?

Before going home, you should be able to answer "YES" to all of the following statements:

✓ I know the names, dosages, side effects and directions for taking my pain medication that have been prescribed.

✓ I know to use relaxation techniques to manage my pain.

✓ I know the importance of distraction techniques to reduce my pain.

✓ I am aware non-pharmacologic therapies that can help to manage my pain.

✓ I know the signs of worsening pain and how to contact my doctor or healthcare provider.

Are there INTERNET resources where I can learn more pain management?

The Joint Commission
www.jointcommission.org

The American Academy of Pain Medicine
www.painmed.org

Preventing Falls

Anne Vanderbilt, Erica Yates & Christina Henrich

Admission to the hospital is a major event with many unknown experiences. One such unexpected event that may occur while you are hospitalized may be a fall. Every year up to 20% of people fall in acute care hospitals across the United States. Injuries from falls may be minor, such as cuts and bruises, or major, such as broken bones and head injuries. Partnering with your bedside nurse can reduce your risk of falling and help you remain safe while in the hospital.

What makes me at risk for falling?

One common myth is that only older adults fall. Although advanced age does increase your risk of falling in general, many other factors may contribute to a fall when you are in the hospital. There are over 600 risk factors for falling. It is important to know your unique risk factors. The following are some things that may increase your risk for falling while hospitalized:

- Certain diagnoses, including stroke, neurological disorders (Multiple Sclerosis, Parkinson's disease), numbness and/or tingling in your feet or legs, heart problems, syncope (feeling of

faintness), orthostatic hypotension (feeling dizzy when you sit up from a lying position), weakness, spasticity and anemia.
- History of falling
- Fear of falling
- The use of a cane, walker, wheelchair, or braces to walk
- Medications that affect your alertness, coordination or need to use the bathroom more frequently
- Specific diagnoses or conditions may cause you to be unsteady because of difficulty with your gait, balance or muscle strength

Additional risk factors are related to the hospital environment itself. The most significant factor is that the hospital is an unfamiliar environment. It is very important that you call for help until you are comfortable and more familiar with your surroundings.

The biggest reason for patient falls is that patients do not want to bother the nursing staff when they want to get out of bed. Contrary to popular belief, nurses do not think that you are bothering them when you put your call light on. Nurses want you to call so you may be assisted out of bed.

How will my bedside nurse know if I'm at risk for falling?

One of the first steps in your hospital experience is a routine nursing admission process conducted by nursing staff members. The purpose of this admission assessment is to learn as much as possible about your individual abilities and needs to best plan your nursing care. The nursing admission process is an opportunity for you, your family and nursing staff members to share important information with each other. Nurses will ask you a lot of questions to help keep you safe from falling. They will perform a "fall risk assessment" using an evidence based tool to categorize your level of fall risk.

Nurses may ask you if you have fallen in the past 12 months and if so, how frequent the falls have occurred and if you were injured. It's important to be honest regarding your fall history even if you were not injured. A prior fall is one of the biggest predictors of future falls. The information you provide about your fall history assists nursing staff to develop an individualized plan of care for you.

What should I do to avoid a fall while I'm in the hospital?

Nurses will continue to ask you questions about falls and assess your condition frequently to determine your level of fall risk. Based on your level of risk, the nurses will develop a plan of care with your participation to help keep you safe. It is important that you understand and participate in the plan. You may want to ask your nurse the following questions:

- Is it ok if I get out of bed by myself?
- Should I call if I want to go to the bathroom?
- Do I need to use a walker or other device?
- Can my family help me out of bed?
- What should I do when I go to testing areas or off the nursing unit?

Your bedside nurse will discuss with you and your loved ones if you are a fall risk and the precautions that are needed to keep you safe from falling.

General fall prevention interventions for everyone include:

- Keeping items within reach such as the call light, telephone, tissues, glasses and TV remote control.
- Turning on the lights prior to getting out of bed, keeping a night-light on in the bathroom and making sure the room is well lit at all times.
- Wearing non-skid footwear. You may choose the hospital-issued slipper socks or bring sturdy slippers or shoes from home.
- Making sure the bed or wheelchair is locked before getting up.

- Reading patient education materials or watching videos about falls.

If you are determined to be at the highest level of risk you may be identified with a symbol such as a yellow wrist band or a special sign outside your room. The purpose of these symbols is to communicate to all caregivers that you require special attention due to your risk of falls.

Some people are high risk for a brief period of time, such as immediately after surgery or a procedure. Other people are high risk at all times due to their underlying disease process or condition. **Most falls in the hospital occur on the way to the bathroom or in the bathroom.** If you are designated as high risk, it is especially important that you partner with your nursing staff. This point cannot be overemphasized as you may feel strong enough to get out of bed by yourself or with a family member, but this is strongly discouraged. Please ask for help.

What should I expect if I am at high risk for falling?

- Your bedside nurse or nursing assistant will instruct you NOT to get out of bed or the chair unassisted. Please call for assistance by using the call light.
- It is suggested that you convey your personal needs while a staff member is in your room. This allows caregivers to attend to any concerns you have immediately.
- With the assistance of a nursing staff member, it is helpful to plan to go to the bathroom in advance of your need. It is important not to wait until the "last minute" as it may be a few minutes until someone can arrive to assist you.
- The nursing staff may develop a schedule to take you to the bathroom to meet your needs during high risk times. This is called a "toileting schedule."

- The nursing staff will assist you in moving about your room as well as the hallways.
- Physical therapists or occupational therapists may be consulted to assess your mobility, strength and flexibility. They will offer a plan to help you move as safely as possible.
- A pharmacist may be consulted to review your medications because certain medications, prescribed at the same time, may contribute to imbalance, weakness and drowsiness.
- If you experience some confusion or problems with your memory while in the hospital the nursing staff will use a variety of strategies to keep you safe. These strategies include:
  ✓ Moving you to a room closer to the nursing station
  ✓ Attaching an alarm to your bed or chair to alert caregivers if you are getting up without assistance
  ✓ Asking a family member to stay with you during meals and vulnerable times, possibly even overnight
  ✓ Assigning you a "sitter or companion" to stay with you during high risk times

Why should I call nursing staff to assist me with getting to and from the bathroom?

There are several reasons you should rely on nursing staff to help you go to and from the bathroom. It reduces your risk for falling and possibly injuring yourself. In addition, it provides nursing staff members an opportunity to evaluate your walking ability. Finally, it serves as a proactive step to prevent the most frequent cause of falls in the hospital.

What if I'm embarrassed to have strangers assist me with toileting needs?

Being hospitalized and requiring the assistance of nursing staff members can be awkward and embarrassing. Those feelings are understandable as adults value their independence and are reluctant to ask for help. Nurses encounter this concern several times a day. They are skilled in balancing your need for independence with the importance of preventing you from falling. Your bedside nurse is dedicated to keeping you safe while you're hospitalized.

Is it OK for family members to assist me to the bathroom without a member of the nursing staff?

Possibly. Always ask your nurse if it is OK for your family member to help you get out of bed. Your condition changes daily, and your family member may need instruction on how to best help you. The nursing staff is very knowledgeable about moving patients safely and efficiently. There are specific techniques that are required to assist patients from different positions and locations. They are the best individuals to assist you to the bathroom. Patients and family members often overestimate their ability to assist with mobility and ambulation needs

In addition, certain medications, such as blood thinners, not only increase your risk for falling, but can also increase risk for injury. Certain conditions may also increase your risk for injury, such as osteoporosis and low blood platelets.

How do I know if I am allowed to get out of bed and walk?

You should be informed of your activity level when you are admitted to the hospital. If you're unsure, ask your bedside nurse or the physician in charge of your care.

How should I request help if I am disappointed or concerned about my nursing care?

Communicate any concerns to your bedside nurse. If this interaction is unsatisfactory, ask to speak to the nurse manager of the nursing unit.

The nurse manager rounds daily and is responsible for the overall care of patients on the nursing unit. When you speak to nursing staff, focus your communication on safety: "I am concerned about my risk for falling, and I think it would be helpful if I were able to be assisted to the toilet more often." Ask for reassurance that your request for timely assistance will be honored, and inquire how your request will be communicated to your other nurses.

What do I need to know to prevent falls and be safe at home?

Before going home, you should be able to answer "YES" to all of the following statements:

- ✓ I know the names, dosages and directions for taking ALL my medications that have been prescribed.
- ✓ I know the side effects of all of my medications, especially those that could make me dizzy or sleepy.
- ✓ I know how to use mobility devices, such as a walker or cane, correctly.
- ✓ I know what changes I need to make to my daily routine to decrease my risk of falling.
- ✓ I have identified a relative, friend or care partner who will check on me regularly.
- ✓ I have access to information about medical alert devices.
- ✓ I know how and when to call 911.
- ✓ I know how to recognize worsening symptoms, such as fever, dizziness and increased weakness.

> ### Are there INTERNET resources where I can learn more preventing falls?
>
> American Association of Retired Persons
> www.aarp.org

Centers for Disease Control and Prevention – STEADI (Stopping, Elderly Accidents, Deaths & Injuries)
www.cdc.gov/steadi

National Institute on Aging
www.nia.nih.gov/health/publication/falls-and-fractures

National Safety Council
www.nsc.org

Veterans Administration National Center for Patient Safety
http://www.patientsafety.va.gov

Promoting Mobility

Nancy Kaser

Moving around in bed and walking in the halls are important to your healing and recovery. Many years ago, bed rest was thought to be the best way to help patients recuperate. Now there is a great deal of research that says moving around and walking aids in recovery, especially for older adults.

Why is activity when you are a patient so important?

Lack of movement or lying in bed for long periods of time can cause many unwanted complications during your hospital stay. Muscle weakness, blood clots and breathing problems are just a few examples. All types of movement are helpful. If you are not able to walk, talk to your caregivers about exercises you can do in bed. Simple activities make a difference. Patients who are as active as possible while hospitalized report that they feel better, are less depressed and require less help once they are discharged from the hospital.

Why is it important for older adults to get out of bed and walk?

Older adults who are independent before entering the hospital can lose their ability to walk while in the hospital. This is because older adults take only 15% of the normal steps they would take at home while they are in the hospital. Older adults are more at risk to the effects of bed rest than younger adults because they have already lost muscle mass due to the normal process of aging.

What are the benefits of walking and moving while recovering in the hospital?

Just as when you are well, there are many benefits from movement and activity during recovery from illness or injury. Moving helps to lessen muscle wasting, improve lung functioning and add to a general sense of well-being. What may be surprising is that physical activity can help to prevent delirium or confusion that sometimes occurs when patients are hospitalized.

How do I become more active when I do not feel well?

Talk with your nurse about any worries you have about getting out of bed and walking by yourself. Your nurse will talk with you about your individual plan for moving, walking, bathing and using the bathroom.

Start slowly. Simple tasks like performing exercises in bed, washing your face, brushing your teeth or sitting at the side of bed may be the best ways to begin moving again. Be out of bed as much as your condition allows. Sit in the chair 3-4 times a day or at mealtimes, and walk in the halls if you are physically able. Nurses understand that this can be difficult when you are not feeling your best, but it is worth the effort. Research has shown that even the very sickest patients improve and have fewer complications when they are moving. It is important that you work with your caregiver team to increase your activity every day.

What do I do if I feel too weak or dizzy to get out of bed?

It is important to promptly report any feeling of weakness or dizziness. This may be due to simply being in bed too long, moving too quickly or the effect of medication or illness. Your caregivers will determine whether or not it is safe for you to be up and about. They also can provide assistance in helping you move around the room or going to the bathroom. Please call for help before getting out of bed. Your safety is very important – put your call light on before you attempt to move! This applies to young and middle-aged individuals as well. You may not think that you are at risk for falling because you are very active and mobile, but being ill and taking certain medications may make you more at risk for falling.

While it is very important to move and spend more time out of bed as you recover, medications and illness may change how much you are able to do before becoming tired. Move and change positions slowly. Sit at the edge of the bed for a few minutes before standing, then stand at the bedside for another minute or two to allow your body to adjust before you begin to walk to the bathroom or ambulate in the hall.

Should I bring my walker to the hospital?

If you use a cane, walker or any device that helps or physically supports you as you walk, this should be communicated to your caregiving team. Most hospitals have basic equipment that you can use while in the hospital. If you do bring your own equipment, make sure it is clearly labeled with your name and contact information.

Are there simple exercises I can do to help me keep my strength while I am recovering in the hospital?

Many of the same exercises you do at home can be modified for use when you are in the hospital. Speak with your nurse, physical therapist or physician before beginning any exercise. Some exercises should be avoided if you have experienced injury or surgery to your knees, hips or shoulders.

Many institutions have instructional videos or handouts that you can refer to as you learn recommended exercises.

Lower body movements that can be done in bed include:

- Ankle pumps – point and flex the foot and toes
- Thigh muscle (quadricep) sets – tighten and relax the thigh muscle
- Butt squeezes (gluteus sets) – tighten and relax the buttock muscles
- Heel slides - from a seated position, bend knee and move heel toward buttocks
- Bridging – lie nearly flat and raise backside off the bed

Upper body exercises to consider include:

- Overhead reach – slowly raise arms straight overhead and then lower them to the bed
- Bicep curls – with the palms of your hands facing upward, bend your elbow and bring your fingers toward your shoulders

Exercises that can be done while seated in the chair include:

- Heel & toe raises – sit straight in chair with feet on floor, then alternate lifting heels and toes off the floor
- Lower leg extension – slowly extend lower leg to straightened position, then return foot to the floor. (Your thigh should remain on the chair.)
- Marching while seated in chair – with knee bent, alternate lifting leg off the seat of the chair.

Is there special equipment that is used to help patients move?

Many patients are familiar with crutches, canes and walkers that are used to assist in mobility. What may be unfamiliar to you are devices used to transfer you safely from one surface to another. A portable lift may be used if you need to move from your bed to a cart to go for a test, or to transfer you from your bed to a chair or chair to the bathroom in the event that you cannot stand or walk safely on your own. Examples of equipment that may be used include an inflatable mattress, a slippery nylon sheet, ceiling lifts or a variety of portable lifts. The goal of safe patient moving equipment is to reduce the incidence of injury to both patients and caregivers.

What do I need to know about going home and staying active?

Before going home, you should be able to answer "YES" to all of the following statements:

✓ I know how much activity is recommended.

✓ I know how to conserve my energy yet participate in exercise.

✓ I am able to perform my prescribed exercises correctly.

✓ I know to stop exercising if I experience any unusual pain or discomfort.

✓ I know when and how to notify my doctor if I have a concern.

Are there INTERNET resources where I can learn more about staying active while in the hospital?

American Academy of Nursing

http://www.aannet.org/immobility-ambulation

Promoting Nutrition

Mary Beth Modic

The word "food" conjures up many images – community, culture and comfort. Food represents some of our fondest memories. Yet, memories of food served when people are hospitalized may not be that remarkable. There are countless cartoons, jokes and get well cards depicting hospital food as overcooked, bland and unappetizing. Moreover, patients and their loved ones frequently complain about the taste and appearance of hospital food, in addition to the arbitrary timing of meals and the lack of feeding assistance to the most vulnerable of patients.

Over the last several years, dietitians, physicians and nurses have been working tirelessly to highlight the importance of serving nutritious and appealing food to patients. Serving meals which look good, taste good and smell good are critical to preventing malnutrition when you are hospitalized.

What is malnutrition?

Malnutrition occurs when there are not enough calories, protein and nutrients to meet the body's needs. Malnutrition can result from a person not eating, sudden illness (acute) or an illness that has lasted longer than six months (chronic). Chronic illnesses that are related to malnutrition include cancer, cystic fibrosis, inflammatory bowel disease, chronic heart and kidney failure, and chronic obstructive pulmonary disease. Treatments and medications can have an impact on nutrition as well. Acute illness malnutrition occurs as a result of increased needs because of infection, surgery or trauma. Malnutrition can increase the time you spend in the hospital because your wounds may not heal as quickly and your muscles may not be as strong. You may find that you are not as able to get up and move around. This can make you more susceptible to constipation, infection or a blood clot, especially if you have had surgery.

How will the doctors and nurses know if I have malnutrition?

When you are admitted to the hospital the nurse will weigh and measure you. She will ask you about:

- Any unintentional weight loss over the past several months
- Poor appetite
- Presence of nausea and vomiting
- Any difficulty chewing or swallowing
- Presence of mouth sores
- Presence of pressure ulcers (also referred to as bed sores)
- Use of enteral (tube feeding) or parenteral nutrition at home (nutrition by vein)

If any of the answers to these questions are yes, a dietitian will be consulted to see you. In addition, blood work will be ordered and reviewed to determine if any of the findings that reflect nutritional status are abnormal. Your dietitian will decide how much protein and calories will be needed to meet your nutritional requirements. Your weight and meal consumption will be monitored every day so that significant weight loss can be prevented. Your dietitian, in collaboration with your physician, may recommend additional nutritional support.

Why is eating a problem in the hospital?

Eating may prove challenging for a number of reasons. The food may be uninviting or be restricted in quantity, texture or flavoring. Illness or certain medications can make you feel nauseated or suppress your appetite. Moreover, meals can be interrupted because of the need for diagnostic testing or surgical procedures.

How do I communicate my special dietary preferences?

It is important to your caregivers that your special cultural or religious dietary practices are honored. Tell your nurse of your dietary preferences. A consult will be placed to the dietitian, who will design a meal plan for you to accommodate your dietary habits and practices.

What do I do if I have no appetite when my meal tray is delivered?

It is not uncommon to have a decrease in appetite when you are in the hospital. Eating is important to your recovery. Try and take a bite or two from everything on your tray. Concentrate on trying to eat the protein that is on your plate. Protein is important in wound healing and infection prevention. Some examples of protein include fish, chicken, legumes, soy and quinoa.

If you are not hungry when your meal tray comes, tell your nurse that you have no appetite. If you wish to eat your tray at a later time, tell you nurse so that your meal can be wrapped, labeled and stored in the refrigerator. Because of food safety concerns, your plate as it is served cannot be left at the bedside. Nutritional supplements or bedtime snacks may be provided to help with your appetite. Asking family to bring in food from home is discouraged because of the potential for food borne illnesses. It may be difficult to maintain food at a correct temperature during transport to the hospital. You may also be placed on a specific diet such as "low sodium" that your family may not know how to prepare.

What should I do if I am not getting enough food to eat?

Speak with your nurse. Arrangements can be made to double the portions of protein and provide more frequent snacks.

How do I get assistance with my meal tray?

Ring your call light when your meal tray arrives, and express your need for assistance. A caregiver will come to assist you with opening cartons and containers and cutting your food. This individual will ensure that you are in a proper position to eat safely, have sufficient light to see your meal, and that your immediate environment is conducive to eating. A caregiver will be informed that you will need assistance since you are too weak or frail to eat.

Encourage family members to visit during meal time. Not only can they offer assistance to you, they can offer companionship while you are eating. They can also advocate for you with your nurse or dietitian if your meal is unsatisfactory.

How will I get nutrition if I cannot eat?

Approaches to improve or maintain nutritional intake are known as nutrition support. These include:

- Oral nutrition support – fortified food or additional snacks
- Enteral tube feeding – the delivery of a nutritionally complete liquid formula that is administered via a tube that is placed in your stomach or small intestine
- Total Parenteral Nutrition, also known as TPN – the delivery of nutrition by an IV placed in your vein.

The decision to provide tube feedings or TPN depends on your condition. You may be ordered nutritional support if you:

- Have experienced a stroke and cannot swallow
- Develop a condition where your gastrointestinal tract (stomach and intestines) is not working
- Had surgery on your throat, esophagus or intestinal tract
- Have not been eating for at least 5 days and may not be eating for a minimum of 5 more days

What is "Room Service"?

Many hospitals have implemented a "Room Service" program similar to hotels. These programs have been created to enhance the patient experience and provide meals that the patient wants to eat. Meals are made to order and are delivered to the patient's room within 30 – 45 minutes from ordering. Modifications to the order may be made if the patient is on a specific diet. In some hospitals that provide this service, family members can order the meals outside of the hospital for their loved ones.

What do I need to know about preventing malnutrition when I go home?

- Malnutrition, particularly in the older adult, is a major reason for readmission to the hospital. Although, you may feel weak and tired upon discharge from the hospital, it is important that you eat even though you may not feel hungry. Here are some tips to help avoid malnutrition:
- Ask family and friends to prepare meals and bring them over as you recover if you live alone. Ask them to bring enough for leftovers so that an extra meal can be frozen for a future meal. Invite them to eat with you so you have conversation and companionship while you eat.
- Contact your church, temple or mosque and let them know that you have just returned from the hospital. Many faith communities provide meals to those recuperating from an illness.

- Strive to eat six small meals a day until your appetite comes back. This may help meet calorie needs when large portions of foods cannot be eaten at one time.
- Eat lean protein, which can be found in lean meat such as chicken, turkey or pork.
- Add peanut butter to whole bread and crackers, celery and fruit slices.
- Consume dairy products as they are also a very good source of protein. Concentrate on low-fat items, such as skim milk, cottage cheese and yogurt.
- Include fiber in your diet by eating fresh fruits and vegetables. Try to follow the saying "eating a rainbow of colors" with lunch and dinner.
- Include whole grains in your diet as well. Eat oatmeal or another whole grain cereal for breakfast.
- Add milkshakes, smoothies and instant breakfast mixes to meals. Investigate the possibility of commercially-prepared nutritional beverages if you are having difficulty eating.
- Keep a record of what you ate at each meal and the time you ate.

What do I need to know about avoiding malnutrition before I go home?

Before going home, you should be able to answer "YES" to all of the following statements:

✓ I know the foods that I should eat to help me recover.

✓ I know the dietary restrictions prescribed by my doctor.

✓ I have family and friends that can help me prepare meals while I recover.

✓ I have an outpatient appointment with a dietitian to help me learn more about my prescribed diet

If you require tube feedings (Enteral Nutrition - EN), you should also answer "YES" to these statements:

✓ I know the name of the tube feeding formula and how many calories are prescribed for 24 hours.

✓ I know how to administer the tube feeding correctly.

✓ I know how to problem-solve difficulties with the feeding pump.

✓ I know how to clean and care for equipment used for feedings.

✓ I know how to care for the feeding tube site.

✓ I know the complications that would require a call to the doctor.

If you require TPN, you should answer "YES" to these statements:

✓ I know the rate and amount of TPN that should be infused over a 24-hour period.

✓ I know how to problem-solve difficulties with the IV pump, including power failure.

✓ I know how to care for the IV catheter and the skin around the insertion site, including catheter repair.

✓ I know how to treat hypoglycemia (low blood sugar).

✓ I know complications that would require a call to the doctor or 911.

Are there INTERNET resources where I can learn more about eating healthfully and nutritional support?

Academy of Nutrition and Dietetics
www.eatright.org

American Diabetes Association
www.diabetes.org

American Heart Association

www.heart.org

American Society of Parenteral and Enteral Nutrition

www.nutrition.org

National Institute on Aging

www.nih.gov/nia

Preventing Pressure Ulcers

Kathleen Hill

Since the time of Florence Nightingale in the 1860s, turning patients in bed and encouraging them to get out of bed if able has been the foundation of pressure ulcer prevention. To decrease your chances of developing a pressure ulcer your nurse will encourage you to get out of bed and move as much as possible, as early as possible. Walking is one of the best ways to prevent pressure ulcers because it relieves pressure and improves circulation to your skin.

How do pressure ulcers happen?

Pressure ulcers, also called bed sores, pressure sores or decubitus ulcers, can occur when your skin is compromised. Examples of how this can happen include when you sit in a chair for too long without shifting your weight or lay in one position for too long. Injury to your skin can also occur when you slide down in the bed or boost yourself up in bed. Even friction from your skin sliding along a sheet can make you prone to injury.

What impact does the hospital environment have on my risk for pressure ulcer?

If you are too sick to get out of bed and walk around, or if you stay in a chair for large portions of the day, you are at greater risk for developing a pressure ulcer. If you are generally unhealthy, unable to think clearly, control your bladder or bowel functions, move yourself without help from others or eat a balanced diet, you will be more prone to developing a pressure ulcer.

Pressure ulcers are most likely to form over bony parts of your body where pressure on your skin and tissue makes it harder for blood to nourish that area. Bony areas of your body at particular risk are those over your lower back and buttocks, elbows and hips. Skin redness that disappears shortly after pressure is relieved is normal. Redness or discoloration that does not go away after pressure is relieved could be a pressure ulcer.

What is considered good skin care?

Your nurse will inspect your skin every day while you are in the hospital. If your nurse finds areas of skin that are red or discolored, she or he may ask you when it appeared and if it is painful or troubling you. Good skin care includes using mild cleansers and moisturizers. If your nurse identifies potential troublesome areas, he or she may place a dressing on the area for added protection.

Your nurse will also consider what you are eating and how much you are eating. If you are not eating well, a dietitian may be consulted. If you have too much moisture on your skin – such as drainage from a surgical wound, loss of bowel or bladder function, or excessive sweat – your skin will be more prone to impairment. Direct contact of urine or stool on your skin is especially problematic. It is important that the skin is cleaned right away. A protective cream may be applied to your skin and absorbent pads may be placed under you to wick moisture away from your skin.

If you must stay in bed, your nurse will assist you to change your position using pillows or other supports to relieve pressure over your bony areas. This change in position happens about every two hours. When you are in a chair or wheelchair, you will be asked to shift your weight every 15 minutes. Most people shift their weight in a chair periodically without even thinking about it. If you are unable to do it on your own, your nurse will assist you.

What are other fundamental principles of pressure ulcer prevention?

There are several strategies for preventing pressure ulcers, including these:

- Avoid lying directly on your hip bone when lying on your side. A 30-degree side-lying position is best. Tuck pillows under one side so that your weight rests on the fleshy part of your buttock instead of your hip bone.
- Keep the head of the bed no more than 30 degrees high to avoid sliding down in the bed. The head of the bed can be raised during meals to prevent choking and lowered one hour after eating.
- Keep your heels off the bed, when lying on your back, by placing a pillow length-wise under your legs from your calf to your ankle. Do NOT place the pillow directly, and only, under your knees as this could reduce blood flow to your lower leg.
- Use pillows or small foam wedges to keep your knees and ankles from touching.
- Keep bed linens as wrinkle-free as possible.

Tips for proper positioning and movement in chairs

If you must stay in a chair or wheelchair:

- Use a seat cushion designed to relieve pressure while sitting at all times. (Avoid donut-shaped cushions, since these reduce blood flow to the tissue.)

- Change position every hour; ask for assistance if you cannot do so by yourself.
- Lift yourself up off the chair every 15 minutes. Depending on your strength, use one of the three methods described below (listed from most to least preferred) and hold the position for at least a slow count of five to 10 seconds:

  1. Place your hands on the arm rest, and lift your body off the chair.

  2. Press your elbow on the arm rest to lift that side of your body off the chair; repeat on opposite side.

  3. Shift your weight by leaning far over to one side and repeat on the opposite side.

- Keep the top of your thighs slightly sloping forward and use pillows or foam cushions between your legs to keep knees and ankles from touching each other.

What will happen if I do develop a pressure ulcer?

There are several signs that a pressure ulcer could be forming. Your skin around the area of pressure may be red, shiny or dark purple (in dark-skinned people, the area might simply become darker than normal). Your skin might be warm to the touch compared with nearby skin. The area may also be swollen or hard and may be painful or lack feeling. If you notice any of these signs, alert your nurse immediately.

Pressure ulcers should always be treated by trained healthcare personnel. Treatment will be tailored to the type of pressure ulcer, its location and your general medical condition. If you have a serious illness or chronic, long-standing conditions, such as heart failure or cancer, the healing process will be more difficult. If you are unable to eat enough healthy foods, or if your body is malnourished, the healing process will take longer.

If you are the visitor of a patient, please encourage your loved one to move. Take a walk. Encourage moving from side to side in the bed. Gently massage lotion on the patient's arms and elbows; offer a back rub with lotion if you and your loved one feel comfortable with this.

What can I do to prevent pressure ulcers when I'm not in the hospital?

Before going home, you should be able to answer "YES" to all of the following statements:

> ✓ I know the importance of getting out of bed or off the couch and moving.
> ✓ I know food to eat that will help me recover.
> ✓ I know my risk of developing a pressure ulcer.

Are there INTERNET resources where I can learn more about pressure ulcer prevention?

Agency for Healthcare Research and Quality:
Preventing Pressure Ulcers in Hospitals
http://www.ahrq.gov/professionals/systems/long-term-care/resources/
pressure-ulcers/pressureulcertoolkit/index.html

The National Pressure Ulcer Advisory Panel
http://www.npuap.org

Teaching Essential Self-Management Skills

Mary Beth Modic

The quote "Teachin' aint talkin' and learnin' ain't listenin'" speaks to the challenges of patient education. Just because your doctor, nurse, pharmacist or therapist told you something, does not mean you understood it or can remember it. Your ability to remember instructions may be affected by your illness, sleep deprivation, medications or worry. Important self-management skills – such as taking medications as prescribed, changing a dressing correctly or following a prescribed diet – may not be remembered completely or accurately. Research has suggested that patients remember between 40 – 80% of information that is provided and less than 50% of what is remembered is accurate!

How do I know what I need to know?

Ask your loved ones to take notes when your caregivers update you about your care, progress and discharge plans. There is so much information that is offered, often in a conversational tone, that it can be unclear what information you need to remember to manage your care at home. Listed below are the major patient education categories that are generally discussed when patients are discharged from the hospital:

- **Taking Medications:** Learn as much as you can about your medications, including the names, dosages, common side effects, when to take each medication and why you need to take each pill, elixir or injection. You will also need to know specific actions to take with specific medications so that the medication can work most effectively. Example instructions you may receive are: "take medication on an empty stomach", "take this medication at bedtime", "avoid eating foods that contain Vitamin K – these include spinach, collard greens and kale."

Your bedside nurse will teach you and explain the need for your medications. In some hospitals, pharmacists may also provide instruction. If you or your loved ones do not understand or are confused about any of your medications, ask your nurse, doctor or pharmacist. Taking your medications as prescribed is ONE of the MOST IMPORTANT things you can do to recover and stay healthy. Dr. C. Everett Koop, the former U.S. Surgeon General, made the following remark about medications, "Drugs don't work in patients who don't take them."

- **Managing Symptoms:** This education refers to activities that you should do to feel better or minimize the common side effects of medications. Suggestions for managing common symptoms that may be associated with your condition or healing will be provided by your doctors and nurses. Examples of common symptoms include fatigue, pain or lack of appetite. Instructions will also include worsening symptoms that require you to notify your doctor or go the Emergency Department. Instructions on whom to call and how to get medical attention 24 hours a day will be included in these instructions. If you do not receive this information, you need to ask, as knowing and understanding this information may prevent you from being readmitted to the hospital.

- **Preventing Complications**: These instructions include strategies you should take to avoid becoming ill or relapsing. They usually focus on following the prescribed diet and level of activity, getting rest, using medical equipment correctly, preventing infections and determining whether your home is safe a place for you to return while you recover. Instructions may include "Avoid eating foods that are high in salt, such as hot dogs and cold cuts," "Get your flu shot," and "Stay away from people who have colds."

- **Keeping your Follow-up Appointments**: Make sure that you have a follow-up appointment after you are discharged. Ask if the appointments can be made before you leave the hospital. This will be one less thing you need to worry about once you are home. It is very very important to keep this appointment(s) so that your recovery and healing can be evaluated by your doctor, nurse practitioner, dietitian or other therapists. Adjustments to your medications or changes in your diet or therapy plan may be made during this visit. If you know that transportation to your doctor's office or hospital is a problem, share this concern with your nurse while you are still in the hospital. It may be possible for a case manager or social worker to arrange transportation.

What is the difference between patient information and patient education?

Patient information is directed at familiarizing you and your loved ones with the plan of care, reducing worry and providing logistics about how and where your care will be delivered.

Examples of patient information include:

- The location where the surgery will be performed – hospital versus ambulatory surgical center
- Directions to the hospital or doctor's office
- A list of blood work that is needed
- Preparations for a successful procedure of test – stop taking a specific medication, don't drink or eat so many hours before the test, etc.
- The length of time you will need to stay in the hospital
- An estimation of when you will be released from the hospital
- A list of the tests and procedures that will be ordered when you are in the hospital
- The schedule for the day of tests, procedures and treatments while you are in the hospital
- Information on whether you will need to consult with other specialists and what type of doctor will come to see you
- Changes in medication therapy to expect while you are in the hospital

Patient education is directed at empowering you and your loved ones to manage your recovery and medical condition correctly and safely at home. The education is tailored specifically to you and your learning needs and requires that you understand the information and can demonstrate the behaviors with a high degree of accuracy.

Examples of patient education content include:

- Stating when and demonstrating how to use an inhaler
- Administering an insulin injection using a pen device
- Changing a wound dressing
- Walking on crutches
- Administering tube feedings
- Selecting foods low in salt from a menu
- Identifying the symptoms of worsening heart failure

- Describing the symptoms of an infection and when you need to call your doctor
- Discussing what actions should be taken when a dose of medication is forgotten

What are survival skills?

These are topics presented while you are in the hospital, which are considered essential in the short term for a safe discharge to home. Survival skills are often chunked or clustered in groups of three to enhance remembering. You may want to ask your doctor or nurse what are the three most important things you need to know in order to recuperate successfully and safely at home.

How will my nurses and doctors know if I understand what has been taught to me before I am discharged?

Your bedside nurse will ask you to repeat in your own words what has just been taught. This technique is called "teach back" and is used to validate that you or your loved ones have understood the teaching. It provides the opportunity for your doctors and nurses to check and reteach if necessary. Example questions include:

- Just so I can be sure that I have presented the information clearly to you, can you tell me why you are taking this medication?
- What should you do if you check your blood sugar and the meter shows a reading of 62?
- When you are changing your dressing, what signs would you be looking for that might indicate an infection?

Your nurse may phrase a "teach back" question this way: "When your wife comes into visit this afternoon, what are you going to tell her we discussed about your heart failure medications?" or "I have given you a lot of information. What are three things you can do to take your medications as your doctor prescribed?"

If you need to learn a skill – such as using an inhaler, changing a dressing or giving yourself an injection – your bedside nurse will observe you and assure you are performing the skill properly and safely. Your nurses, doctors and therapists may wish to observe you performing the skill several times before you are discharged.

In addition to verbal instructions, caregivers might provide you with written pamphlets, booklets, DVDs and trusted internet sites to reinforce the teaching that was given. Many hospitals also have excellent patient education programs that are shown via television in you room. You and your loved ones may be instructed to watch these programs as well.

If you feel overwhelmed or have difficulty remembering instructions, share these concerns with nurses, doctors and other caregivers who are teaching you. It may be determined that you need home healthcare or therapy delivered to you in your home.

What is self-management?

Self-management describes the level of involvement a patient exhibits in managing a chronic condition or disease. Behaviors that are associated with effective self- management include learning more about one's condition, participating in self-monitoring activities, making informed decisions and taking necessary action to prevent complications or worsening health. Patients with chronic diseases such as arthritis, cancer, diabetes, heart disease, heart failure, high blood pressure, inflammatory bowel disease or neurological conditions realize that learning about a diagnosis in a doctor's office, clinic or hospital hardly prepares them to live or cope with their condition. Ongoing learning, practice and making adjustments to the plan of care are all components of living with a chronic condition.

Learning about your condition:

- Ask questions of your doctor, nurse practitioner, pharmacist, dietitian or therapist
- Discuss your options, concerns and goals with your doctor, nurse practitioner, pharmacist, dietitian or therapist
- Attend community based educational sessions provided by healthcare professionals who are experts on the topic being presented
- Read books and patient education materials
- Talk to family, friends and other people with the same condition
- Search the internet and seek trusted or credible websites

Participating in self-monitoring activities required for your condition includes the following:

- Weighing yourself daily
- Measuring your fluid intake daily
- Checking your blood sugar as frequently as recommended
- Checking your blood pressure
- Tracking the number of steps you take daily
- Measuring the amount of carbohydrates you are eating at each meal
- Taking your temperature

Making informed decisions includes:

- Deciding what your priorities are
- Setting realistic goals with your doctor or other healthcare providers
- Deciding what treatments you do and do not want in collaboration with your family and caregiving team

Taking necessary actions includes:

- Reviewing and changing your health related behaviors including eating healthfully, being physically active, maintaining a healthy weight, not smoking and coping effectively with problems such as frustration, anger, fear and isolation
- Seeking support from healthcare professionals and clergy
- Socializing with family and friends who bring you joy, love and comfort
- Making changes to the way you spend your time
- Engaging in activities that are important to you

What is the difference between patient compliance and adherence?

The word compliance implies that the patient is passive and was not involved in the creation of the medical plan or healthy lifestyle plan. Compliance describes how well a patient follows medical advice, primarily how closely the patient follows the directions for taking the medication as prescribed. When patients do not follow the prescribed therapies, they may be viewed as uncooperative, incompetent or unable to follow directions by members of the caregiving team. It is a very negative label and does not address why the patient did not follow the medical advice. Non-compliant is equivalent to earning an "F" in good patient behavior. You may be anxious to see your doctor, nurse practitioner or therapist for a follow-up visit because you fear a stern lecture or scolding for not following the instructions.

There are many reasons why patients do not follow medical advice. Possible explanations include:

- Unable to understand the therapy
- Unable to know what to do if they fall off track
- The plan is too complicated
- Medication is too expensive
- Life is too stressful

- Experiences unwanted/intolerable side effects
- Sees no reason to continue treatment

The word adherence suggests that the patient assumes an active role in his or her care and collaborates in the plan of care. This results in patients being more confident and successful in managing their illness and taking their medications.

What are other reasons patients may not follow their doctor's advice?

Other challenges that can affect how well patients are able to follow the instructions is how long the activity is required. If it means checking your blood sugar or that of your child at least four times a day, every day, seven days a week, 365 days a year, you can feel overwhelmed and may feel that this expectation is not manageable. Adhering to a diet that is low in salt, fat, sugar, free of gluten and high in fiber may seem as appetizing as eating cardboard. Taking multiple medications that make you feel sluggish, constantly hungry, or gain weight may make you reluctant to take them as you think you feel better without them.

Additional barriers that can prove challenging include instructions that conflict with your cultural or religious beliefs. Even more disheartening is that while you understand all of the information, you just can't figure out how you are going to remember to take all of your medications, perform your exercises and get enough sleep. You are reluctant to share this information for worry that your caregivers will label you "noncompliant."

What can I do to avoid the label non-compliant?

Speak with your caregiving team about your worries and concerns. Perhaps you are a bus driver or a teacher and taking a diuretic (water pill) is unrealistic for you. Perhaps you are worried about taking 8 pills, three times a day. Are there other medications that may yield the same results and require you to take 5 or 6 pills twice a day?

Maybe the cost of your prescriptions seems high so you plan to cut the pills in half to save money. This can cause problems if your doctor thinks you are taking the medicine correctly and then prescribes a higher dose. Your caregivers can not help you if you do not share your personal story or preferences. Let them know of your reluctance to take so many medications restrict foods that are the mainstay of your diet or change your dressing. The Joint Commission has created a Speak Up™ campaign that reinforces the importance of being proactive when it comes to learning about your illness and what you can do to have a smooth recovery.

This chapter has described the importance of learning about your medications, managing symptoms and preventing complications. It has highlighted the difference between education you should receive prior to being discharged from the hospital and education you need to manage a chronic disease if you have one.

Before going home, you should be able to answer "YES" to all of the following statements:

✓ I have received education about my medications.

✓ I have received education about managing symptoms.

✓ I have received education about preventing complications.

✓ I have received education about who to call or what to do if I am experiencing serious side effects from my medications or complications.

✓ I have received written instructions about how to care for myself at home.

✓ I have received referrals for ongoing education and therapies if necessary.

Are there INTERNET resources where I can learn more about self-management practices?

Health Literacy Resources
http://www.aafp.org/online/en/home/clinical/publichealth/ptpops/healthliteraryresources.html

Indian Health Service
www.ihs.org

Joint Commission
http://www.jointcommission.org /630.792.5000

MedlinePlus Comprehensive information
from the National Institutes of Health
http://www.nlm.nih.gov/medlineplus/aboutmedlineplus.html

Preparing for Discharge and Care Transitions

Dianna Copley

Members of your caregiving team will begin discussing your discharge at the time of your admission. It may seem peculiar that your doctors and nurses are discussing your discharge after you were just admitted, but there are many members of the team who need to be involved to help ensure a SAFE discharge.

What is discharge planning?

According to the Centers for Medicare and Medicaid (CMS), discharge planning is a "process of determining what needs you have to move safely from one level of care to another." You may be able to go home with a family member who will watch over you and help you recuperate, or you may need home healthcare services because you require additional nursing care or physical therapy services. You may not be able to return home right away and need to recuperate in a rehabilitation facility (rehab), skilled nursing facility (SNF) or long-term acute care facility (LTAC). Comprehensive discharge planning can prevent you from being readmitted to the hospital, help you recover and provide you with education to take your medication and use medical equipment correctly.

Why does my doctor want to get me out of the hospital so soon after I was admitted?

Being hospitalized carries many risks. Staying in the hospital longer than is medically necessary can increase the risk of infections, medication errors, depression and loss of independence. Your doctor wants to get you home as soon as you are physically stable and fit for discharge.

 By planning for your discharge early in the hospital admission, concerns such as insurance coverage, home healthcare services and transportation can be addressed so that your discharge is a smooth and safe transition. If you require care in a rehab, SNF or an LTAC, planning early will also allow you and your family to make a decision about the facility that will best meet your needs.

What issues are considered in a discharge plan?

A discharge plan should include details of the type of care that is needed and whether it will be provided at home or at another facility. Other elements of the plan include the education, medical equipment and additional help required to provide safe care at home.

Specific care issues that are evaluated to determine whether you can be discharged home or require care at nursing or rehab facility include:

Health status:

- Ability to perform personal care – bathing, toileting, grooming, dressing independently
- Ability to walk without falling or use walking aids correctly
- Ability to fill prescriptions and take medications as prescribed

- Ability to eat, prepare meals or administer tube feedings accurately
- Ability to manage symptoms effectively
- Ability to keep follow-up appointments
- Ability to call for help or seek medical attention if condition worsens

Home environment:

- Clean home and in good repair
- Ease of access to bedrooms and bathrooms
- Free of hazards – no area rugs, electrical cords or excessive clutter
- Adequately heated and cooled
- Adequate space to accommodate need for medical equipment – hospital bed, walker, commode, shower chair, oxygen

Availability of family/friends:

- Physically, cognitively and emotionally able to support you
- Informed of care needs
- Demonstrated competence in performing skills necessary to assist with care – inject medication, change dressings, administer tube feedings, perform blood glucose testing
- Informed of follow-up care needs – appointments, additional testing, home healthcare services, signs of worsening condition*
  *List is not intended to be comprehensive.

How do I learn about what I need to do at home?

Discharge instructions will be provided to you by your caregiving team and are generally reviewed with you by your bedside nurse. If you do not understand all of the instructions, share this with your doctor or bedside nurse. Research has demonstrated that 40% of patients over 65 have experienced a medication error at home and 18% of patients have been readmitted to the hospital because they did not fully understand the instructions. It is important to ask questions. The only 'bad question' is an unasked question. If you have complex discharge needs, a case manager will be consulted and you may be assigned a care coordinator to help you navigate your care while you recuperate.

Should I go the emergency room if I feel sick after I get home?

Your caregiving team will review the reasons to call your physician or conditions that require you to go to the emergency room or call 911 after you are discharged home. Reasons to call 911 or go to the emergency room are:

- Problems with breathing, such as choking or trouble breathing
- Changes in your mental status, such as new confusion, passing out, inability to speak, see, walk, move, or weakness and drooping on one side of your body
- Chest pain or pressure
- Heavy bleeding, including blood when you cough, throw up or have a bowel movement
- Intense and uncontrollable pain
- If you are having thoughts of harming yourself or someone else

If you believe your condition may be able to wait, call your physician and seek medical advice. Many patients will be provided with an 'on call nurse' phone number at discharge, which they can call for questions.

If you do go to the emergency room or call 911, it may be helpful to have a family member gather your recent discharge materials, especially if you are visiting a different hospital's emergency department.

What is a Case Manager?

Case Managers are social workers or registered nurses who identify healthcare needs, living arrangements and social support for patients with complex social and financial needs. Their involvement in your care often ends at discharge.

What is a Care Coordinator?

Care Coordinators are different than case managers. Care coordinators are assigned to patients with complex healthcare needs, such as diabetes and heart failure. Your care coordinator will work closely with you to identify resources specific to your needs, enhance communication among your providers and serve as an additional support for you. Care coordinators ultimately want to help improve your functional abilities, advocate for you and reduce the amount of time you spend in and at the hospital.

How do I get help at home to help me recover?

Many of the services that are provided in the hospital can also be provided in your home. Your caregiving team will help determine which home healthcare services you need to be continued at home, such as physical therapy, occupational therapy, and skilled nursing care. Skilled nursing services can include education, home safety instructions, wound care and infusion therapy. Your case manager will help to arrange these services based on your insurance coverage and will work with you in selecting an agency.

While your case manager can help to arrange certain services – such as your medications being delivered in the hospital before you are discharged and having equipment delivered to your home – some services are not included in home care. Home care does not routinely include laundry, cleaning and making meals. Talk with your caregiving team if you have concerns about how you will provide these services for yourself, especially if you will not have family and friends available to help you.

Are there community resources to help me with meals or transportation?

Many communities offer a variety of resources, especially to senior citizens, for meal assistance and transportation needs. Your registered nurse can ask the social worker to discuss these resources with you.

Will my insurance cover home healthcare?

Every insurance company coverage differs, which is why discharge planning begins early in the hospitalization. After you are at home, your home health agency should disclose to you if a service or material will not be covered before providing it. If you have a question about coverage, please ask your case manager before discharge or your home health agency after discharge.

How do I get the equipment I need to care for my loved one at home?

Certain equipment, such as wheelchairs, walkers, and hospital beds, are called 'durable medical equipment' and can be ordered by your doctor. Some healthcare insurance will cover some or all of the cost of durable medical equipment that is necessary. Delivery of this equipment may be able to be arranged before you are discharged, which your case manager will help with. If equipment needs to be picked up or is not covered and you need time to decide if you want to purchase it, your doctor can write a prescription for durable medical equipment.

Who can help me as I feel overwhelmed about caring for myself when I go home?

If you have concerns about caring for yourself, please speak up and let your doctor or nurse know before the day of discharge. Home health services can be arranged for certain conditions. Your diagnosis, physical health and healthcare needs will determine what type of facility will be the best to help you heal and recover from your illness or surgery.

What is the difference between a skilled nursing facility, a rehabilitation facility and a long-term acute care facility?

Skilled Nursing Facilities (SNF) provide care for patients who are ready for discharge from the hospital, but have additional care needs that cannot be managed at home. Examples of care needs include tracheostomy care, wound care, physical or occupational therapy, and intravenous (IV) antibiotics.

Rehabilitation (Rehab) facilities accept patients from the hospital who require additional rehabilitation services that would be best met at a facility instead of at home based on the recommendations of Physical & Occupational Therapy (PT/OT).

Long-Term Acute Care (LTAC) facilities generally accept patients from the intensive care unit (ICU) who require specialized services, including ventilators and complex wound care. Patients often require rehabilitation services after discharge from the LTAC.

No matter which type of facility is recommended to you at discharge, you and your loved ones will be offered a choice in selecting the facility. As facilities may be full at the time of your discharge, it is a good idea to have some alternative choices selected.

What should I look for in a rehabilitation facility?

If you are having a surgery that will require rehabilitation services afterward, discuss this with your surgeon to determine if you can pre-select a rehab facility. Factors to consider when selecting a facility include your insurance coverage, distance from your home and if the facility can provide the exact type of care you will need.

Questions you should ask when choosing a rehab are:

✓ Can they provide information for the patients who have required similar care to mine?

✓ Will I see the same one or two physical therapists?

✓ How often is therapy provided?

✓ How long are the therapy sessions?

✓ Will a doctor oversee my care?

✓ Will the facility educate me and my family members before my discharge?

How do I know that the nursing home will take good care of me or my loved one?

Selecting a nursing home can be an overwhelming decision, particularly if it has to be made unexpectedly. Ask people you trust, such as friends, work colleagues or clergy from your faith community, for recommendations. Some doctors visit SNFs, so you may want to consider a certain nursing home that your primary care physician visits if maintaining that relationship is important to you.

Another important consideration is the location of the nursing home in relation to your home or distance from family and friends who will visit you. Your case manager will provide you with names of facilities that are located in your preferred geographical area. Family members or friends should tour the facilities prior to your discharge.

What follow up appointments and testing are needed?

Your discharge instructions will include the appointments and testing that are scheduled after your discharge. Often, these appointments can be made before you leave the hospital. Clarify the location of the post hospital visit, since your doctor may see patients at many locations throughout your city.

Make sure to ask if there are any special instructions regarding any laboratory studies before you leave the hospital.

What should I do if I cannot get an appointment within the time period that the doctor instructed?

Make sure that the provider you are trying to see is aware that you were recently discharged from the hospital and that you were instructed to make a follow-up appointment within a certain time frame. Contact your care coordinator, if you were assigned one, and ask for assistance in obtaining an appointment. If you have been provided with a phone number for a 24-hour nurse line, call and ask for advice and assistance.

What can I do to prevent being readmitted to the hospital after going home?

Before going home, you should be able to answer "YES" to all of the following statements:

- ✓ I know the names, dosages and directions for ALL of my medications that have been prescribed.
- ✓ I have a prescription for all medications.
- ✓ I have a prescription for all of the medical equipment I will need.
- ✓ I know which medications I should STOP taking.
- ✓ I know what foods and drinks I should consume to promote my health.
- ✓ I know the restrictions on driving and returning to work.
- ✓ I know when to follow up with my physician.
- ✓ I have the necessary referrals (such as physical therapy, diabetic education or nutrition therapy).
- ✓ I know the home healthcare services that will be provided and know the name of the agency providing services.
- ✓ I know who to call if my condition worsens or I have a question.

✓ I have received a referral to a social worker or case manager if I have financial or social concerns that will prevent me from obtaining medications, oxygen or other home supplies.

Knowing and understanding your discharge plan will help prevent you from being readmitted. Once you return home, update your medication list to include any new prescriptions. If you elected to create or update your advance directives while in the hospital, put these documents with the rest of your important healthcare paperwork.

How can I be prepared should I need to return to the hospital in the future?

Consider the information you were provided in the beginning of this book. Information including your updated medication list, advance directives ("living will" or "durable power of attorney for healthcare") and including information on why you were hospitalized should be kept together. Do not begin any new medications, herbals or supplements without first discussing these with your primary healthcare provider.

Are there INTERNET resources where I can learn more about caring for myself after discharge?

Aging and Disability Resource Center
www.adrc-tac.acl.gov

Centers for Medicare and Medicaid Services
www.cms.gov

Eldercare Locator
www.eldercare.gov

Family Caregiver Alliance – National Center on Caregiving
www.caregiver.org

National Long-Term Care Ombudsman Resource Center
http://ltcombudsman.org

National Patient Safety Foundation
www.npsf.org/download/SafetyAsYouGo.pdf

Nursing Home Compare
www.medicare.gov/nursinghomecompare

Supporting End of Life Care

Deborah Klein & Diana Karius

I t is not easy to be a patient or the loved one of someone who is experiencing a progressive life limiting illness. The anticipation of death is
fraught with fear and anxiety. Nurses and physicians who bear witness at
the end of life have a deep understanding of the human experience of fear
and suffering and are tremendously skilled in providing comfort at the end
of life. Most people wish to be at home at the end of their life surrounded
by their loved ones. Palliative care and hospice care are two specialties that
help patients achieve this wish.

What is palliative care?

Palliative care focuses on managing the symptoms as well as addressing
the emotional, spiritual and psychosocial distress that are associated with a
serious illness. Palliative care is provided by a number of caregivers including physicians, nurses, social workers, case managers, music therapists,
nutritionists, art therapists and chaplains. This ensemble of caregivers
manage all the needs you or your family have as you confront a serious illness. Goals of care will be developed with you and your loved ones so that
your wishes will be honored. Special attention is dedicated to maintaining
your quality of life. Not all patients who are seen by palliative caregivers

are at the end of their life journey; end of life care is one small component of palliative care.

How are family members included in care decisions?

Once the palliative care team is consulted, a family conference is scheduled to make certain that you and your loved ones understand what is happening and to discuss your goals of care. Anyone can request a conference including you, your loved one or a member of your caregiving team. Your physician, bedside nurse and social worker are the caregiving team routinely present at a family meeting.

What is hospice care?

Hospice is a care philosophy that is an available option to patients when life expectancy is six months or less. Hospice care utilizes the expertise of physicians, nurses, social workers, case managers, bereavement counselors, chaplains and volunteers to provide compassionate and holistic care. Hospice care is focused on comfort at the end of a person's life. Hospice care does not speed up or slow down the dying process, but supports the natural dying process to make the patient as comfortable as possible. Hospice care is available regardless of age or ability to pay.

Where is hospice care provided?

Hospice care is usually provided in the patient's home. It can also be provided at a free-standing hospice center, hospital or a nursing facility if the patient's care needs exceed the family's ability to care for the patient at home. Hospice services are available to patients with any type of illness.

When does a person need hospice care?

Enrollment in hospice care is strongly encouraged as soon as the life expectancy has changed to less than six months. This allows you and your loved ones to establish relationships with the new team so they can fully appreciate your needs and wants. They also teach your family members, who will be the primary caregivers, the skills they need to care for you.

What services does hospice provide?

In addition to empathic and expert caregivers, hospice also provides needed medications, supplies and medical equipment. The hospice caregiving team is alert to subtle changes in the patient and are skilled in communicating these changes and what they mean to family members. Hospice also provides bereavement counseling to surviving family and friends.

Why is it important to select a family spokesperson?

Patients in the hospital are often asked to select a spokesperson who will be responsible for informing and updating your loved ones about the plan of care and any changes that may be mutually agreed upon by you and your physician. The person you select should be someone you trust. Your caregiver team will communicate with you and your spokesperson about the treatment plan, your response to treatment and address any concerns.

What are advance directives?

Advance directives are legal documents that provide instructions about who should oversee your medical treatment and what your end-of-life wishes are, in case you are unable to speak for yourself. These documents may include a healthcare power of attorney paper, living will, Do Not Resuscitate (DNR) order and/or organ and tissue donor registry enrollment form.

If you already have these documents, please be sure to bring a copy of each one to the hospital. It is helpful to have these papers made if you have not done so. If you do not have them but would like to fill them out, please have a member of your caregiving team contact the social worker. The Social Worker can bring the papers to you, help you to fill them out and ensure that they become part of your medical record. These papers will help your caregiving team follow your wishes. This will decrease the stress on your loved ones because they will not have to make difficult choices.

What does "Do Not Resuscitate" (DNR) mean?

A Do Not Resuscitate (DNR) order indicates that a person – usually with a terminal illness or other serious medical condition – has decided not to have cardiopulmonary resuscitation (CPR) attempted in the event his or her heart or breathing stops. Often a DNR order is written by a physician after discussing the burdens and benefits of CPR with you or your surrogate decision maker. DNR order definitions may vary by state, but are usually divided into three categories:

1. Your caregiver team provides all therapies to keep you alive including CPR, medications, and electrical therapies (i.e. defibrillation of the heart).

2. Your caregiver team provides only those therapies selected by you or your surrogate decision maker, i.e. defibrillation of the heart, but not placing a breathing tube (intubation).

3. Your caregiver team provides comfort care before, during and after the time your heart or breathing stops. You receive medication to relieve symptoms such as pain. This option is usually recommended for those who are at the end of their life since no treatment will change the course of the disease.

A DNR order may be changed at any time by speaking to a member of the caregiving team.

What is comfort care?

When death is near or certain the caregiving team will concentrate on providing comfort care. This type of care is directed at managing pain, breathlessness and anxiety. Every effort is made to ensure a "good death." A good death means that the patient is not afraid, not in pain, not short of breath and his or her wishes have been honored.

How will my wishes be honored as I approach my final days of life?

Your caregiving team is dedicated to providing end of life care that honors your wishes as well as incorporates the religious and cultural practices that are important to you. Your bedside nurse will be intimately involved in caring for and advocating your needs. Your nurse will envelop your loved ones in your care as well, by informing them of physical changes, asking them to assist with bathing and other physical care (if they wish) and providing privacy.

Can my pet be brought into the hospital or hospice center?

Pets are important members of the family. Different institutions may have certain requirements to allowing pet visitation. If this is important to you, please let your caregiving team know so they can inquire and facilitate as much as is possible.

What are the physical signs of dying?

All dying experiences are unique and influenced by many factors, such as the particular illness and the types of medications being taken. There are some physical changes that are fairly common. For some, this process may take weeks; for others, only a few days or hours.

For most dying persons, activity decreases significantly in the final days and hours of life. They speak and move less and may not respond to questions or show little interest in their surroundings. They have little, if any, desire to eat or drink. Your loved one may sometimes be fully awake and at other times not responsive. Periods of restlessness are common. Often before death, people will lapse into a coma or become unresponsive.

You should always act as if the dying person is aware of what is going on and is able to hear and understand voices. In fact, hearing is one of the last senses to remain before death. You can continue to talk to your loved one or touch him or her if you wish.

It is not unusual for dying persons to experience sensory changes. Sometimes they misperceive a sound or get confused about some physical object in the room. They might hear the wind blow but think someone is crying or see a lamp in the corner and think someone is standing there. These types of misperceptions are called illusions. They are misunderstandings of something that is actually in their surroundings.

Dying persons may hear voices that you cannot hear, see things that you cannot see or feel things that you are unable to touch or feel. This can be comforting to the dying person. These happenings may be very upsetting to you. Try not to ask your loved one to stop or try to correct the situation. Try to keep conversations open and honest. Share old memories, and allow your loved one to share stories about his or her life. Allow your loved one to participate in these conversations as much as able.

The dying person may feel cool to touch because there is less blood flowing to the hands and feet. As death approaches, skin color is likely to change from the normal tone to a duller, darker, grayish hue. The fingernail beds may also become bluish in color or darker.

When a person is just hours from death, breathing often changes from a normal rate and rhythm to a new pattern of several rapid breaths followed by a period of no breathing. Fluid can start to build up in the lungs. This may cause a rattling sound as they breathe. This breathing sound is often distressing to loved ones, but it is not an indication of pain or suffering.

It is difficult when a loved one is ready to let go, but the opportunity to say goodbye is a final gift of love. Since hearing is the last of the five senses to be lost, it is important to speak in a normal tone of voice, say whatever you need to say to him or her and assure your loved one that it is okay to "let go." This may be as simple as saying "I love you".

Can I be an organ donor?

If it is acceptable in your culture and possible, please discuss donating your organs with your loved ones in advance. There are thousands of people who are on a transplant list waiting for an organ. You have the opportunity to save a life of a stranger with your gift of generosity. Giving the "Gift of Life" may lighten the grief of your family, knowing that there is a part of you allowing a man, woman or child to have another chance at life.

Who will help my loved ones after I die?

There are many people who can help you through this time of profound loss and grief. Caring for a loved one who is dying can be mentally, physically and spiritually exhausting. Once your loved one dies, you may feel a wide range of emotions, including a sense of relief that your loved one is no longer suffering or afraid. It is important to know what resources are available to help you. Your hospice nurse and social worker will be able to guide you toward the resources that will most helpful to you.

Be gentle with yourself. Accept offers of help. Do things that bring you comfort.

Are there INTERNET resources where I can learn more about hospice or palliative care?

American Hospice Foundation
www.americanhospice.org

Center to Advance Palliative Care
www.getpalliativecare.org

Centers for Medicare & Medicaid Services
www.medicare.gov

Department of Veterans Affairs
www.va.gov

National Hospice and Palliative Care Organization
www.nhpco.org

National Institute of Health: National Institute on Aging
http://www.nia.nih.gov

Visiting Nurse Associations of America
www.vnaa.org /202.384.1420

Part Three:

Partnering with your Caregivers to Manage Your Chronic Medical Conditions

"Somewhere, somehow, at some time in the past, courageous nurses determined these skills, learned them, fought for the right to use them, refined them, and taught them to other nurses. All nurses have an obligation to remember that part of nursing's past, and to keep their own skills in pace with new opportunities for nursing into the next century."

Hilldegard Peplau, RN

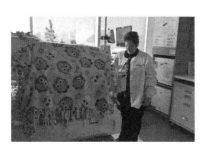
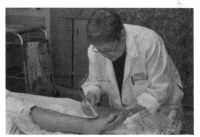
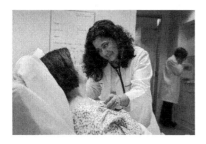
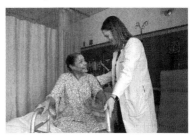

Alzheimer's Disease

Jeanne Sorrell

A patient may be hospitalized for an illness or surgery but at the same time be experiencing memory problems caused by Alzheimer's or another type of dementia. If you have a loved one with dementia who is admitted to the hospital, you can be an advocate for him or her to help make the hospitalization as comfortable as possible. You are the expert in knowing what comforts and what causes distress in your loved one. Your caregiving team will rely on you for recommendations on how to best provide care.

This chapter is written as a guide for you, the reader. Rather than describing the care nursing provides, the intention is to help you guide the nursing caregivers in the most appropriate care for your loved one. The information pertains to you visiting your loved one in the hospital. Although the information refers to "he," it is equally relevant for women with dementia. If your family member has mild dementia, he may want to read the information himself.

What can I do to advocate for my loved one?

It is important that you inform nursing staff exactly how the dementia is affecting your loved one's ability to remember and follow directions. There is a wide range of severity of dementia in different persons. Many persons with early Alzheimer's can function so well that the nurses and other hospital staff may not realize that dementia is present. They may not understand why your family member is not responding to requests as expected. On the other hand, if the staff sees on the admission information that your family member has Alzheimer's, they may assume that he is unable to communicate, even though his memory is minimally affected. Thus, one of the most important things that you can do is communicate clearly with the nursing staff so that they know your family member's capabilities and limitations.

What will happen if my loved one has to be taken to the emergency department?

It is likely that your loved one may be admitted to the hospital through the emergency department. The fast-paced, noisy and unfamiliar environment of the emergency department is likely to create anxiety for any patient, but it is especially frightening for someone with Alzheimer's, who may not be able to understand what is happening to him and why strangers keep poking him. It is important for you not to leave your loved one alone. You can be very helpful to both him and the staff by helping to decrease his anxiety and facilitate communication.

The following activities can be very helpful for your loved one in the emergency department:

- Provide continuous cues about what is happening and reassurance that your loved one is going to be safe and well cared for.
- Guide the staff in approaches to communication that have worked well in the past, such as asking simple "yes" and "no" questions, making eye contact and allowing adequate time to respond.

- Encourage the staff to describe what they are doing, why they are doing it and that it will be finished soon.
- Make sure that the staff do not talk about your loved one as if he was not in the room. You can politely remind them that he can understand directions if they are communicated carefully.
- Communicate your loved one's history to the nursing staff to assist with diagnosis and treatment.
- Pay attention to changing levels of consciousness. Increased signs of confusion or delirium can signal acute changes in his illness.
- Watch for behaviors such as grimacing, restlessness or anxiety that may signal that he is in pain, and communicate this to the nurses.

What will happen to my loved one during hospitalization?

All patients benefit from feeling secure and comfortable, but for a person with Alzheimer's, feeling secure can make the difference between cooperative interactions and difficult behaviors. The trauma of the illness that preceded hospitalization, the strange new environment, the disrupted daily routine and the influence of medications can all be factors that lead to increased anxiety and confusion.

How can I help manage the hospital environment to reduce confusion in my loved one?

You can help the nursing staff understand what type of environment is likely to help calm your loved one and make him feel more comfortable. Most patients who have Alzheimer's feel more secure in a simple, uncluttered, quiet environment with routine activities. One of the most helpful interventions is to maintain a consistent, structured, predictable atmosphere.

- When admission is planned, ask the admitting nurse if it is possible to have a private room away from the noise of ice machines, people congregating to talk, etc.

- Eliminate distracting noises such as the radio, TV or loud conversation. It is helpful to keep the television off unless your loved one wants to watch it.

- Avoid clutter in the room. It can increase confusion, agitation and the risk of falls.

- Work with the nursing staff to provide a consistent, predictable routine, as change is often difficult. Ask if the same nurses and nursing assistants can provide care whenever possible.

- Collaborate with nurses to schedule rest periods during the day. Post "Patient Resting" or "Do Not Disturb" signs on the door of the room.

- Monitor the effect of visitors, and limit them as needed to maintain rest.

- Bring in security objects from home – such as a favorite pillow or quilt – and place pictures of friends and family members where they can be easily seen. If your loved one always carries a purse or some other object, it can usually be arranged for this to be kept in the bed with the patient.

- When your loved one is taken from the nursing unit for diagnostic tests, it is helpful if someone from the unit staff can accompany him. The strange and fast-paced environment of X-ray and other diagnostic areas can be confusing and frightening for someone with Alzheimer's.

How do I make sure that the nursing staff knows how to communicate with my loved one?

Your loved one has probably become comfortable with ways of communicating at home, but now in the hospital he is faced with communicating with so many strangers that it may seem overwhelming. You can be helpful to the nursing staff by sharing information about communication techniques that you have found effective. The following ideas may be helpful to share with them:

- Always begin by identifying yourself and calling the patient's name. Maintain eye contact, and speak slowly and calmly with short, simple sentences. Use concrete language.
- Avoid using the in-room intercom. Hearing a voice without seeing the person may be confusing and even frightening.
- Find out if a patient wears glasses, a hearing aid or dentures, and place them nearby the patient. Sometimes, however, a patient may feel more comfortable without them.
- Do not ask orientation questions, such as "Where are you?" once a patient's inability to answer this is established. Most patients are very aware of their inability to remember and become distressed when they know they cannot answer appropriately.
- Reality orientation is not helpful. Instead of repeating information like "Today is…," use memory aids, such as a large sign with the date. Label objects, such as "closet" or "bathroom."
- Give the patient adequate time to respond to your question. It may take as long as 20 seconds. If you need to repeat your question, phrase it exactly the same way.
- Give directions as simply as possible, and only give one direction at a time. Use gestures to help understanding, such as an upward hand gesture with the direction "stand up."
- Humor can be helpful. If you are cheerful and laughing, a patient will sense this and is likely to follow your lead.

Can the nurses adjust the timing of when they feed or bathe my loved one?

You may have established a daily routine for your loved one at home that he feels comfortable with. In the hospital, however, he is suddenly expected to adapt to the daily routines of nursing staff, such as when to eat, bathe and sleep, with frequent interruptions for vital sign measurements, medications and various treatments. Ask the nursing staff if some of the routines on the unit can be adjusted to fit better with your loved one's routine.

Help the staff understand that allowing patients with Alzheimer's to follow routines they did at home is very important. When routines are altered, it requires the patient to plan a new way of doing it, which creates anxiety. Persons with Alzheimer's learn through repetition, so if they have to concentrate harder on an activity, the task becomes more difficult.

What can I do to make sure my loved one eats while in the hospital?

Eating is an important daily activity at home or in the hospital. However, many of the hospital routines that relate to eating may seem very different from what your loved one is used to at home. He may not be able to fill out a menu request, so you can help him select nutritious foods that he likes. Also, the large number of food choices may seem overwhelming so you can help him narrow down the options. If your loved one needs special finger foods, cups with lids or broad-handled utensils, be sure and inform the nursing staff. They will arrange for you to talk to a hospital dietitian.

The hospital food may be delivered on a tray with unfamiliar plates, cartons and wrappings, so your loved one may not recognize bread wrapped in cellophane, milk in a container or silverware in a paper envelope. Make sure that he has help in setting up his tray when you are not with him.

Persons with late-stage Alzheimer's may be able to chew, but need frequent reminders to swallow. They may also need reminding to drink enough fluids during the day, as adequate fluids are very important. You might want to bring in a drinking container that your loved one uses at home. Some patients hesitate to drink enough fluid because they worry about incontinence, so make sure that he knows that someone will help him with toileting needs.

Sometimes patients do not eat adequate amounts of food because they worry about not being able to pay for it. If you find this is the case with your loved one, reassure him that his Medicare or insurance will take care of the cost. It might be helpful to give him something tangible like a punch card or ticket that states he is entitled to the food.

What is the best way to manage my loved one's bathing and toileting needs?

Some patients with Alzheimer's are afraid of the water when they take a bath or shower at home. In the hospital, bathing may be an especially frightening experience. Talk with the nursing staff about how to make the bathing process as comfortable as possible for your loved one. It may be helpful to arrange the bath at the same time as at home. If he refuses when the staff suggest the bath, they may want to wait about 20 minutes and then ask again, as this gives him some sense of control. Staff should encourage him to do as much as possible for himself; if they need to assist, they should give the bath slowly and gently and explain what they are doing at each step. If the process is agitating him, it is better to stop.

Nursing staff should use the same procedure with oral care that your loved one does at home. With guidance, he may be able to brush his teeth by himself.

The nurses will tell you whether your loved one is allowed to walk to the bathroom or use the bedside commode. He may have been more independent in toileting at home and may be upset by a change in procedure that limits this independence in the hospital. Help him understand that this is temporary until he gets stronger. Incontinence is understandably upsetting for him, so make sure that he is placed on a regular toileting schedule. If he is allowed to walk to the bathroom, make sure that there is a clear pathway. It may be helpful to place a picture or a written sign on the bathroom door as a reminder.

Nursing staff often ask patients each shift if they have had a bowel movement, but persons with Alzheimer's may not remember and the question might upset them. To avoid this, make sure that bowel movements are recorded regularly. Observe for signs of constipation, such as abdominal discomfort or grimacing.

How will my loved one's pain be managed?

Hospitalized patients who have Alzheimer's may have pain from chronic illness, surgery or some other procedures done while they are in the hospital. These patients are sometimes not treated for pain in a timely manner because changes in behavior are thought to be from the dementia process when they are actually related to pain. You can help nursing staff understand when your loved one needs pain medication or another intervention. Some hospitals have nurses who specialize in pain management; a nurse on the unit could ask for a consult for your family member.

You can be an advocate for your loved one by reminding the nursing staff to consider the following:

- Watch for signs of discomfort, even though a patient might not verbally complain. Observe facial expressions and body language
- Moaning, shouting, restlessness or sudden worsening of behavior may indicate pain. A refusal to do activities that have become routine may also signal pain.
- Take all signs of pain seriously.
- Confusion can make assessment of pain difficult. However, even confused patients can be asked if they have pain. They may not be able to describe it or provide a number to rate the extent of the pain, but they can often point to a location of the pain.

What can be done to keep my loved one safe?

You have probably implemented measures at home to help ensure the safety of your loved one, but the hospital often presents new challenges. Discuss with the nursing staff any concerns you have about safety. Some of the following are ideas to consider if your loved one wanders:

- Make sure the nursing staff knows your loved one wanders.
- Share with the nursing staff how you have managed wandering at home.
- Ask for a room where the staff can watch your loved one carefully and that is away from the stairs or an elevator.
- Provide a picture of your loved one to place at the nursing station so that all employees will know who to look for if he wanders off the unit.

The tendency to wander may be increased when someone is stressed, anxious or in pain, so it is helpful to anticipate that. Make sure that pain is assessed and treated. If your loved one can walk, plan regular walks. Also, keep his travel bag and street clothes out of sight.

Other safety ideas to consider:

- It may not be safe to raise the side rails on the bed because your loved one may try to climb over them and fall.
- Make sure a pathway to the bathroom is lighted at night.
- If your loved one has any kind of tubes inserted, be creative in working with staff to protect the tubes from being pulled out accidentally.

What is delirium?

Delirium is a state of increased confusion that can come on rapidly. As many as 25% of patients with Alzheimer's develop delirium during hospitalization. If your loved one's behavior suddenly changes and he seems to have extra confusion, agitation or hallucinations, where he sees or hears imaginary things, he may be experiencing a state of delirium. Physical stressors such as pneumonia, wound infections, urinary tract infections or fluid imbalance can lead to delirium. If you observe that your loved one's confusion seems to be worsening, of if he is experiencing hallucinations, it is very important to notify nursing staff so that they can intervene to treat the possible cause of the delirium.

What is a catastrophic reaction?

The term "catastrophic reaction" is often used for a sudden emotional outburst from a person with Alzheimer's. The person may feel overwhelmed and thus overreact to real or imagined stressful events. It may be related to past events and memories or tasks and instructions being too complicated, such as being asked to perform a task beyond one's abilities. An environment that is too stimulating, with too many strangers and too many questions being asked at one time, can trigger a catastrophic reaction. Fatigue can also bring on this type of emotional outburst, as can irritable, impatient staff.

If your loved one has had a catastrophic reaction in the past, help the nursing staff understand what triggers these events so that they can try to avoid them. If your loved one has a catastrophic reaction for the first time in the hospital, it is important to consider the following:

- Remain calm, use a low tone of voice and do not argue with him.
- Discontinue the activity that was in process and restart it later.
- If possible, move him to a quieter area.
- Do not force or restrain him.
- Offer reassurance and try distracting him.

To try to prevent a catastrophic reaction:

- Use simple communication techniques and instructions with step-by-step directions.
- Maintain a simple, structured and secure environment with routine activities and schedules.
- Introduce and implement new treatments slowly.
- Make sure that body language is calm and nonthreatening.
- Limit choices so that a selection is made between two items instead of multiple ones.
- Build in rest periods.

Research has shown that people with Alzheimer's or other dementias are more likely than other older adults to be hospitalized, especially for conditions such as pneumonia, urinary tract infections, worsening heart failure or dehydration. These conditions may be treated without hospitalization if they are caught early enough, so it is important that someone monitors your loved one's health and reports any unusual changes, such as fever, fatigue, pain, shortness of breath or burning with urination. However, sometimes it is difficult to observe these changes at an early state.

If your loved one does need to be hospitalized, it is important not to blame yourself. You have a great deal of knowledge that can be extremely helpful to share with staff in ensuring that your loved one has a comfortable hospital stay. Your presence at the loved one's bedside can be very calming. But it is important also to take care of yourself. Being the caretaker for a person with dementia can be exhausting, even when he is hospitalized. Make sure that you balance your time with your loved one in the hospital with your own rest so that you can be ready to help him return to his previous environment after discharge.

What are some INTERNET resources that can help me understand and care for my loved one with Alzheimer's disease?

Alzheimer's Association
http://www.alz.org/

Alzheimer's Foundation of America
http://www.alzfdn.org/

Alzheimers.gov
http://www.alzheimers.gov/

Cancer

Diana Karius & Christina Colvin

This chapter will discuss the care you should expect if you are admitted to the hospital with a cancer diagnosis. Having an understanding of what to expect is a large part of helping you feel safer and more in control of your care.

What tests will be performed every day?

Although daily weights and vital signs are not "tests," their findings present your caregivers with important information. Your weight will be measured daily so that the doses of medications can be adjusted. Many medications are dosed according to weight.

Your vital signs, which include assessing your temperature, heart rate, breathing and blood pressure, will be monitored at regular intervals around the clock to help detect any changes in your condition.

Nurses will check your blood counts daily or as frequently as needed. You may be awakened to have your blood drawn as the results will direct the medications or care that you will receive during the rest of the day. It might also be necessary to draw blood samples at various other times of the day.

Blood can be drawn from your arm, or you might have a special device, such as a tube or catheter placed for blood draws and treatment. If you already have a device, please let your medical team know.

Cancer diagnoses and treatments can have an effect on your blood cells. For this reason, your caregiving team will regularly monitor your blood counts in a series of tests referred to as a Complete Blood Count (CBC). The three main types of blood cells are:

- **Red Blood Cells (RBCs):** These cells make your blood red in color and make up almost half of your blood. If these are low, you may feel tired and short of breath. Anemia is a condition referred to when your RBCs are low.
- **White Blood Cells (WBCs):** These cells help prevent and fight infection. There are many types of WBCs. Neutrophils are a particular type of WBC that kill harmful bacteria and are your first line of defense against infection. Checking the number of neutrophils in the WBC is especially important for determining your risk of infection and your body's ability to protect itself. Neutropenia is a condition referred to when your WBCs are low.
- **Platelets:** These cells help stop bleeding and repair damage to your blood vessels. Thrombocytopenia is a condition referred to when your platelet count is low. When your platelet count is low, you may have bleeding from your gums or nose. Women may experience heavier than usual menstrual periods. You may see random bruising, without injury. If you do cut yourself, you may bleed more than usual; for this reason, electric razors are recommended for shaving. When your platelets are low, your caregivers may remind you not to do things such as shaving with a non-electric razor or blowing your nose.

What will be done to treat my low blood count?

Blood or blood product transfusions, such as red blood cells and platelets, may be needed during your stay. The possibility of receiving a blood transfusion concerns some patients who worry about contracting AIDS or other infectious diseases from the blood. All blood products are tested for any possible contamination, and transfusions are monitored to ensure patient safety. Your medical team can explain what type of transfusion you require and why.

How will my nurse help me take care of myself?

When you are feeling tired or have low energy, you may not feel up to bathing or brushing your teeth. Your nurse or nursing assistant will assist you in bathing and performing mouth care if you are feeling too weak. Bathing is very important to help prevent infections. Supplies for bathing are usually provided; however, feel free to bring your own.

Mouth care is a very important daily routine. Keeping your mouth clean decreases the risk of mouth sores and infection. Sometimes special mouth care is needed. Your bedside nurse will provide instructions. Otherwise, continue your normal mouth care routine, which should include brushing your teeth at least twice a day.

How will my pain be managed?

If you are on pain medications that control your pain at home, please bring that information with you to the hospital so that those medications and dosages can be ordered for you. Keeping your pain under control is an important goal for your caregiving team, and you will be assessed frequently to determine if your pain is managed.

How do I stay active in the hospital?

During your hospital stay, it is extremely important to stay active. The more active you are, the stronger your body will be. This will aid you in your recovery. Walking in the halls several times a day is strongly encouraged. Some areas may have exercise equipment available for use during your hospital stay, such as, treadmills, exercise bikes, etc. Even getting out of bed and sitting in a chair is helpful to keep your body strong, prevent skin breakdown, prevent falls and aid in digestion.

Do I need to be on a special diet?

Some medications may require you to change or eliminate certain foods from your diet. Your caregiver team will determine the diet appropriate for your care. There are no approved "anti-cancer" diets. Eating a well-balanced diet, maintaining your current weight and drinking plenty of fluids are recommended. A dietician may be consulted to address your concerns about diet and weight. They may recommend liquid nutrition drinks, if needed.

How can I minimize my risk for developing an infection?

Avoiding people with colds and flu is a very important step to take to help prevent infection. Request that any friends or loved ones who have been ill refrain from visiting you until they are well. All caregivers and visitors should clean their hands with soap and water or an alcohol-based hand rub upon entering your room. Caregivers should also clean their hands with soap and water or an alcohol-based hand rub before and after caring for you. Some sinks and hand rub dispensers are located outside of patient rooms; it is OK to ask your caregivers or visitors if they cleaned their hands before entering your room. Many hospitals have alcohol-based hand rubs available for patients to clean their hands, however it is best to wash your hands with soap and water before eating and especially after you have gone to the bathroom.

How will I know if I have an infection?

Your caregiving team is committed to preventing infections. It is a goal that every hospital in the United States shares. Occasionally, patients may develop an infection while in the hospital. Symptoms of infection include all or some of the following:

- Fever, chills, sweating
- Sore throat or mouth sores
- Coughing
- Difficulty breathing
- Stomach pain
- Frequent urination or burning during urination
- Severe diarrhea

What are possible side effects of my treatment?

Depending on what type of cancer you have, you may receive one or a combination of different types of treatment. Treatment can include chemotherapy, surgery, radiation or other types of medication. Your medical team will decide and discuss with you which treatment or treatments would be most effective for your type of cancer. Regardless of your treatment, you should always feel comfortable to ask questions. It is OK to ask questions until you understand information that is unclear or confusing. Since this is a very stressful time, having a loved one or friend with you during any care discussions is helpful. Some people find that taking notes during these discussions is also helpful.

Your caregiving team is dedicated to helping you cope with the side effects from any of these treatments, which may include nausea/vomiting, diarrhea/constipation and fatigue. Medication can be given on a regular basis or as needed for relief from side effects. If your side effects are not managed as expected by the medication provided, it is OK to request additional or different medication or an alternative treatment. Although many side effects can be managed by medications, there are many other options available as well. Many hospitals provide services such as, guided imagery, music therapy, pet therapy, art therapy, massage and Reiki to assist in the management of side effects and anxiety.

What are some strategies for helping me cope with my diagnosis?

Facing the reality of a serious illness can be overwhelming and difficult. Complex and unfamiliar medication plans, chemotherapy and radiation treatments, and separation from family and friends can increase your anxiety. Most people find these changes challenging. Consider what has been helpful and unhelpful to you in the past when dealing with stressful or difficult situations. Here are some positive coping strategies:

- Stay connected with friends and family. Having loved ones or friends visit or call you can be very reassuring. Share your feelings about what is happening to you, and allow your friends and family to comfort you.
- Be an active partner in your treatment plan. Ask questions, voice concerns, and seek clarification when explanations from members of your caregiving team are unclear to you.
- Ask for help when you think you need it. Allow your family and friends to offer assistance with meals, transportation or childcare.
- Focus on things you can control. Let go of things you can't change or control, and concentrate on doing things that will help distract you or connect you with family and friends.
- Surround yourself with people who bring you joy and happiness. Minimize the time you spend with individuals who drain your energy or make you feel discouraged or sad.
- Focus on what needs to be done in the present moment. It is easy to get overwhelmed if you think about all of your responsibilities and relationships and what you need to do while receiving treatment.

- Speak with you minister, priest, imam or rabbi. Seeking spiritual counsel can provide a great deal of consolation.
- Talk with your social worker about your fears and concerns. They may also have information on programs and support groups that can provide assistance.
- Accept your reactions and your own natural pace of coping. Acknowledge your feelings about your diagnosis and treatment, and give yourself time to adjust. There is no timetable for coping with a cancer diagnosis.
- Expect the unexpected. Remind yourself that there are events you cannot control. Few things will happen exactly as expected. Plan for delays, setbacks and surprises.
- Learn as much as you can about your disease and its treatments. This can help you feel more in control and more comfortable with the plan ahead.

What do I tell my young children about my cancer?

It is important to be honest and consider what your child might be able to understand. Don't be afraid to use the word "cancer." In addition, consider this advice:

- Tell or show where the disease is on your body. If you don't talk to your children, they may create their own ideas, which could be even more frightening.
- Prepare your children for any physical changes you might undergo during your treatment.
- Let them know who will continue to take care of them.
- Reassure them that they cannot catch the disease and that they did not do anything to cause the disease.
- Encourage your children to take part in your care, such as having them bring you a glass of water, a pillow or a book. It is helpful for the child to feel involved.

- Urge your children to express their feelings. When helping your children cope with your diagnosis, it's almost impossible to be prepared for every situation. Sometimes you may not know what to say. This is normal and okay.
- Illness and hospitalization can be overwhelming and disruptive, but it doesn't change the fact that you know your children best.
- Trust your sense of how to best support your children during this difficult time.

Adult children may benefit from working with your cancer social worker. The social worker can assist them with information on financial support, advance directives/care planning and the importance of choosing a legal spokesperson to help with decision making in the future. The social worker can also make recommendations for support groups and services.

What do I need to know about managing my symptoms at home?

It is likely that your medication was modified while you were in the hospital. Be sure you have a good understanding of any changes to how your cancer/symptoms are being managed.

Before going home, you should be able to answer "YES" to all of the following statements:

   ✓ I know the names, dosages and directions for taking ALL my medications that have been prescribed.
   ✓ I know how to take my medications to minimize their side effects.
   ✓ I know what to do if I miss a dose of my medication
   ✓ I have a plan for obtaining and refilling my medication.
   ✓ I know how to reduce my risk for getting an infection.
   ✓ I know how to manage my symptoms with medication, rest or diet.

✓ I know when and whom to call about signs and symptoms of an infection, shortness of breath, dizziness, lightheadedness, unexplained bleeding, ongoing fatigue, confusion, nausea, vomiting or pain that is uncontrolled.

✓ I know how to care for my IV access (PICC line, Mediport, Hickman®, Broviac®).

✓ I know how to balance rest with activity to conserve energy.

✓ I know what resources to use to help cope with my diagnosis and treatment.

Are there INTERNET resources where I can learn more about cancer?

American Cancer Society
www.cancer.org

Cancer Support Community
www.cancersupportcommunity.org

cancer.net
www.cancer.net

Caring Bridge
www.caringbridge.org

Chemocare.com®
www.chemocare.com

National Cancer Institute (NCI)
www.cancer.gov

Depression

Jeanne Sorrell

Mood disorders such as depression affect millions of people. If you are one of those people, it is important to think about how being in the hospital may affect your care. It is also important to think about what you can do to help ensure that nurses and other healthcare staff understand that you are feeling anxious and depressed so that they can offer you support.

Depression is a condition that can affect you in different ways.

- You may not have thought much about depression and consider yourself a happy person. But then you are admitted to the hospital for surgery or treatment of some illness like stroke or cancer. As you think about how the illness has changed your life, you realize that you suddenly feel depressed.
- Or you have had a diagnosis of clinical depression and have been receiving medication that has helped. Now, as you are hospitalized for surgery or an illness, you realize that the medication you have been using is no longer working well.

- Or perhaps you have been taking medication at home for clinical depression and it is no longer controlling your symptoms. You feel hopeless and have thoughts about hurting yourself or others. You realize that you need to be admitted to the hospital in order to have your depression evaluated so that you can get a new treatment plan.

Whichever of the conditions above applies to you, there are things that will be helpful to know in relation to having depression while you are hospitalized. Anyone who comes into the hospital for treatment may feel frightened and anxious. With depression, you may have other symptoms, such as difficulty concentrating, lack of pleasure in things that would usually make you happy, feelings of worthlessness and hopelessness, not wanting to see friends and families, and even headaches, gastrointestinal problems, or heart palpitations. If you are experiencing any of these symptoms, you should talk about them to your nurse or doctor so that they can help you.

What should I do before I am admitted to the hospital for an illness or surgery?

You may feel anxious or overwhelmed at the thought of being admitted to the hospital. It is a good idea to ask a family member or friend to go with you and help you through the process of filling out paperwork and getting settled in your room. If possible, you or they should call ahead of time to find out about the hospital's rules and procedures and ask about what items you should bring with you. Information about visiting hours and telephone access will also be helpful so that you know you will have contact with friends and family who are important for support.

What will happen once I'm in the hospital?

Once you are settled in your room, a nurse and other hospital staff will help explain the treatment plan that the caregiving team has for you. It is important that you know what medications you have been taking, as well as the amounts and times that you take them. It is good to bring along a written list of these medications, since it is sometimes hard to remember them when you are under stress. If you have been taking medications for depression, it is very important to tell the nurse or doctor about them, how long you have been taking them and how you have been feeling while taking the medication.

Although psychological testing is not a usual part of hospitalization for surgery or medical disorders, sometimes your doctor may feel that you should be evaluated for anxiety or depression during your hospital stay. In this case, there are a variety of assessment tools that could be used. One tool that you may be asked to complete is the Hospital Anxiety and Depression Scale (HADS). This tool has been tested in research studies and found to be a valid assessment of anxiety and depression. It only takes about 5 minutes to complete and can help staff know when you may need extra support for your anxiety or depression. Assessment with this tool works best if you just answer the questions according to your first impression, rather than thinking about them too long. Try to remember that completing this tool should not make you anxious. It is designed to give your healthcare staff insight into how best to support you during your hospitalization.

What should I know about the medications prescribed for depression?

If you were diagnosed with depression before your admission, you may already be taking antidepressants. If you are diagnosed with depression after your admission, your doctor may start you on these medications. There are also other types of medication related to depression that may be ordered for you in the hospital. Some of these are anxiety-reducing medications or sleeping pills.

Sometimes these medications can help you get rid of symptoms of depression in a few weeks or months, but you may need to continue them for a longer time. This treatment only works, however, if you continue to take the medications as long as they are prescribed for you. If you stop taking them on your own, your symptoms of depression may return. At some point, your doctor may start to decrease the medication. This is usually done gradually so that your symptoms don't flare up again. Some people with recurrent depression may need antidepressants for several years or even the rest of their lives.

With all medications ordered for you in the hospital, be sure you know whether the nurse is going to give them to you routinely or whether you need to ask for them. Some medications are listed as "prn," which means that they are only given when you need them. For these medications, be sure and ask the nurse for them as soon as you feel that you need them.

You should know what each medication is supposed to do for you and specific side effects of the medication. Medications for depression sometimes affect people differently according to their age, medical problem, other medications, etc. Be sure and tell the nurse or doctor if the medication does not seem to be affecting you the way you think it should. Always report any concerns you have to a nurse or doctor.

When should I go to a hospital to be treated for depression?

If you have been treated for depression outside the hospital, there may be a time when you find that the medication is not controlling your symptoms and that the symptoms have become more severe. If this happens, your doctor may want you to be admitted to the hospital so that you can receive treatment to better control your symptoms. Remember that a mood disorder is an illness that needs treatment, like diabetes or heart disease, and sometimes it is better to be treated in the hospital.

Being admitted to the hospital for this type of treatment may seem frightening, but the controlled environment of the hospital can help you become more stable and feel better. Treatment in the hospital can create a safe place for you to be while waiting for your severe symptoms to pass. No one outside of your close family needs to know about the hospitalization if you prefer that. Being admitted to the hospital for any reason is between you and your admitting doctor. It is the patient who determines who will be notified about the admission.

A decision for hospitalization for depression may be appropriate when you need a safe place in which to receive intensive treatment until your symptoms stabilize. If you are undergoing major changes in your treatment plan for depression, your doctor may want you to be in the hospital so that you will have close supervision. Also, you may have been feeling stable at home on your medication, but then your symptoms become more severe. You may have thoughts of harming yourself or others or you may feel too ill to eat, bathe or sleep properly and you realize that your treatment just isn't working any more. Situations that indicate that you may need to seek help for possible hospitalization include:

- Feelings of wanting to harm yourself or others
- Feeling hopeless and that you don't want to go on living
- Feelings of agitation or rage
- Feeling trapped
- Having wide mood swings
- Having little control over your emotions, such as frequent sobbing
- Hallucinations where you see or hear things that are not present
- Delusions where you believe things that aren't true
- Problems with alcohol or drugs
- Inability to eat or sleep or eating or sleeping too much
- Gaining or losing weight large amounts of weight unintentionally
- Disinterest in social contact
- Unable to care for yourself or your family because you cannot make yourself get out of bed to bathe and dress

- You have tried different therapies and medications for depression and still have bad symptoms that significantly interferes with your life

What can I expect to happen when I'm admitted to the hospital for depression?

When you are admitted to the hospital specifically for treatment of depression, you will have somewhat different experiences than when you are admitted for a physical illness or surgery. One of the first things that will happen is that you will be evaluated by a psychiatrist in order to identify a treatment plan that meets your specific needs. Other mental health professionals may also work with you, such as psychiatric nurses, a clinical psychologist, social worker and therapists that focus on activity and rehabilitation. It may take as long as a week after your admission to the hospital before your actual treatment plan is finalized. This period of time may be needed to enable the healthcare staff to assess you carefully, make a correct diagnosis and develop the best possible treatment plan.

Part of your treatment plan may be to participate in individual sessions with a therapist, but group therapy and family therapy may also be used during your hospital stay. You will probably receive one or more psychiatric medicines. Some of these may be medications that you have taken at home, but you may also be given new medications. It is important for you to let the healthcare team know how these medications are affecting you and whether they seem to be controlling the symptoms that brought you to the hospital.

While you are in the hospital, there may be important educational opportunities that will help you learn more about your illness. Nurses and other healthcare personnel may teach you about such topics as:

- What it means to suffer from depression

- How the illness typically progresses
- Various treatment options
- Purpose and side effects of medication

It is good for you to participate in these educational sessions, as they can help you gain insight into your illness and the different types of treatment.

You may be concerned about whether your insurance will pay for your hospitalization and how much and how long it will cover your care in the hospital. Hospital personnel will take care of getting approval from your insurance company for your stay and will probably tell you if they encounter any problems related to your coverage. If you are unsure of whether your hospital stay is covered, however, be sure to ask to talk with someone in the billing office about your insurance.

It is important for you to let your caregivers know how you want your family members to communicate with you and your caregivers. There are privacy regulations in the hospital that limit the kind of information that can be communicated about you to family members who call the nurses to see how you are. These regulations are to ensure that the details of your treatment in the hospital remain confidential, so make sure that your family members know what kind of information can be provided by the nursing staff. It is a good idea to identify one family member to communicate regularly with the nursing and medical staff so that the hospital personnel will know that you are comfortable with them talking to this person on your behalf. This family member can then share whatever information you agree to with other family members.

You should be aware of your rights as a patient. You have the right to be completely informed about all tests and treatments you will be receiving, including their risks and benefits. You have the right to refuse any tests or treatments that you feel are unnecessary or unsafe. In addition, you may refuse to participate in any experimental treatment or training sessions involving students or observers. If you have been admitted to the hospital voluntarily, you also have the right to sign yourself back out. Before you make this decision, however, you should discuss it with your nurse and doctor. They can explain to you how leaving the hospital may affect your treatment plan. If the hospital staff believes that you are a danger to yourself or others, they will want you to stay in the hospital. The key is to be open and honest with those caring for you so that they can address your questions and concerns and help you feel safe.

What do I need to know in order to go home?

Whether your treatment for depression in the hospital lasts for a few days or a few weeks, you may be anxious to be discharged and return to your home. Be sure that you take the time to have the hospital staff carefully explain to you what your post-hospital treatment will be. Make sure that you know what medications you should be taking and what new prescriptions you may need. It is difficult to remember all of this when you probably are already stressed, so be sure that you write down the details of all of your post-hospitalization care that will be needed. Find out if a follow-up appointment has been made for you with your doctor, and make sure that you know who to call in case of an emergency.

Your doctor may recommend a day-treatment program after discharge in an outpatient clinic or community mental health center. This type of program can help you continue with some of the treatments that you had during your hospitalization.

How do I plan for the future?

It is important for you to realize that depression is a chronic illness, so it is good to have a plan of action in case you ever need to be hospitalized again for depression. Keep a current list of the following:

- Your doctor's name and contact information

- Contact information for friends, family or support group members
- A list of all medications that you take
- A list of any allergies
- A list of any medications you cannot take
- Your insurance information
- The name of the hospital where you prefer to be treated

One of the most important things to remember is that you are not alone in dealing with depression. In addition to your friends and family who can provide support, there are many community agencies that can be helpful. One important community resource is the Depression and Bipolar Support Alliance (DBSA). This organization has a wealth of information on depression that can be helpful to you.

DBSA has hundreds of support groups across the United States to provide people with depression, as well as their loved ones, practical ways to cope with depression and work toward wellness. Research has shown that people who participate in DBSA groups for more than a year are less likely to be hospitalized for their mood disorder. People who participate in these groups have mood disorders and experiences similar to yours. Sharing your experiences with them in a safe and confidential environment can be helpful in learning coping skills and gaining confidence in ways to lead a happy and productive life.

Before going home, you should be able to answer "YES" to all of the following statements:

✓ I know the names, dosages and directions for taking ALL my medications that have been prescribed.
✓ I know how to take my medications to minimize their side effects.
✓ I know what to do if I miss a dose of my medication.
✓ I know the importance of keeping my follow-up appointments.

✓ I know how and when to use relaxation techniques.

✓ I know the names of support groups that may be helpful and how to contact them.

✓ I know how to increase my physical activity to help with my depression.

✓ I know the foods I should eat to promote physical well- being.

✓ I know the benefits of designing a sleep schedule to reduce stress.

✓ I know the importance of prioritizing responsibilities, such as housework, paying bills and errands, to reduce feelings of being overwhelmed.

✓ I know the benefits of keeping a diary to track my medications, moods and any important changes in my lifestyle.

✓ I realize the necessity of asking for help from family and friends when I need it.

Are there INTERNET resources where I can learn more about depression?

Centers for Disease Control and Prevention
www.CDC.gov

Depression and Bipolar Support Alliance
http://www.dbsalliance.org

National Alliance on Mental Illness
http://www.nami.org

National Institute of Mental Health
http://www.nimh.nih.gov/health/topics/depression/index.shtml

Diabetes

Mary Beth Modic

When you have diabetes, being admitted to the hospital can be very unsettling. Most of the time, your diabetes is not the main reason that you are admitted to the hospital. As a result, your doctors and nurses may worry more about your heart condition, infection or recovery from your surgery – the reason that you were admitted – than your diabetes. You are the expert in managing your diabetes, and it is very important that you tell your doctors and nurses how you manage your diabetes at home.

When you are sick your glucoses can fluctuate more than they do when you are at home. It is important to share with your nurse and doctor your diabetes care routine at home. It is not always possible to receive the same brand of insulin you are taking at home. However, you will be prescribed insulin that acts in the same way as the insulin you take at home. If you are taking insulin, it is important to be aware of the time your blood sugar is checked, your meal is delivered and the time your insulin is administered. These should all be within a 30-minute time period.

Factors that can contribute to blood sugar fluctuations in the hospital include:

- Missed meals or not being permitted to eat in preparation for an operation or procedure
- Certain medications
- Insulin that is not coordinated with your blood sugar check and meal
- Insulin dosing error (too much or too little insulin is prescribed or given)
- Worsening physical condition

Why is it important to control my blood sugar in the hospital?

High glucose levels slow the healing process and increase the risk of infection. Managing diabetes in the hospital reduces illness, shortens hospital stays and even lowers the risk of death. Diabetes control in the hospital improves a person's chances of having the best possible medical outcome.

How do I convey my expectations about my diabetes management to my doctors and nurses?

When you are being admitted to the hospital, SPEAK UP. Tell your doctor and nurse how important it is to you to have your blood sugar under control. Tell them about your daily efforts to eat healthfully, be active, monitor your blood sugars and take your medications/insulin as prescribed. It is also a good idea to share with all of your caregivers how you manage blood sugar swings and what daily care practices you use to manage your diabetes well.

If managing your diabetes is difficult for you, share those concerns with your caregivers as well. Diabetes requires time, knowledge and support. There is no vacation from managing your diabetes. A referral to a social worker, case manager or certified diabetes educator may help with your concerns.

What important self-care practices regarding my diabetes management should I share with my nurse?

It's important to provide your nurse information about the following self-care practices:

- Frequency of blood sugar checks
- Medication/insulin to control blood sugars
- Meal Plan – how many carbohydrates you eat at each meal
- Exercise Regimen at home
- Coping Strategies – relaxation techniques, yoga, meditation, prayer, journaling, support, etc.

What information should I share about the challenges I encounter in managing my diabetes?

Your caregivers will want to know the following:

- Frequency of blood sugars higher than your target blood sugar
- Frequency of low blood sugars
- Symptoms of low blood sugar
- Any diabetes complications – nerve pain, high blood pressure, kidney disease, vision changes, etc.

How will I know what is going on with me while I am in the hospital?

The doctors and nurses want you to be very informed about what therapies, treatments or tests are being done to help you recover from your illness or surgery. At the change of shift, the nurse who has cared for you will introduce you and your loved one to the new nurse who will be assuming your care. At this time, your nurse will be "reporting" or "handing off" to the next nurse what took place during the past shift and what is the plan for the next shift. This "report" is usually done at the bedside so that you can participate by asking questions or clarifying the plan. With regard to your diabetes management, you want the nurses to communicate with each other the following:

- Your type of diabetes
- Blood sugar values and trends – whether your blood sugar has been high just at bedtime or low after lunch or within target range
- What action was taken if you had a high or low blood sugar
- A possible explanation of what could have caused the high or low blood sugar – a certain medication, a missed meal, a missed dose of insulin, eating food brought in from home, etc.
- Your prescribed diet
- Amount of meal consumed
- Tests/procedures that require you to not eat food (referred to as "NPO") and the plan for your basal insulin
- Discharge plan

If you are admitted to a teaching hospital, your doctor may visit you accompanied by several other people. They may be doctors in training (known as residents or fellows), your bedside nurse, a nurse practitioner or physician assistant, a pharmacist, a respiratory therapist or a dietitian. Ask your doctor to introduce you to all these individuals. Your doctor will discuss with you the results of the tests you have undergone in the hospital as well as changes in medication, diet or activity. Further testing that may be necessary. Your doctor will be able to identify when you should be well enough to go home or that you may need to recuperate in a rehab facility until you gain sufficient strength to go home.

Many hospitals have developed ways of writing the plan down and communicating that to you and your loved ones. Ask your bedside nurse how this is done at your hospital.

I take oral medication for my diabetes at home. Will I be prescribed those medications in the hospital?

As a general rule, most patients' oral diabetes medications are stopped in the hospital. This is because meals are often unpredictable or interrupted. Often you will be prescribed insulin while in the hospital so that your blood sugars can be controlled since you are no longer taking your oral diabetes medications. Ask your doctor or nurse how your diabetes will be controlled in the hospital.

What should I ask my doctor about my diabetes management if I need surgery?

Ask your doctor if your medication/insulin regimen will be changed or modified the day before and day of surgery. You should ask your surgeon about the possibility of being the very first surgical case of the day. You should bring an accurate list of all your medications that you are taking, but most importantly you should be able to describe your diabetes medication/insulin regimen, monitoring practices and dietary and physical activity habits. Your regimen will be altered while in the hospital because your body will be stressed as a result of surgery. In addition, your meal consumption and physical activity will be reduced while you are recovering. These are all factors that will change the diabetes regimen you use at home.

It is very important that your doctors and nurses be aware of what you do at home to manage your diabetes. They will use this information to help you recuperate from surgery and reintroduce your home regimen as you recover.

What should I expect when my meal is held for a test?

Your mealtime insulin will not be given because you have not eaten any carbohydrates that would cause your blood sugar to rise. However, if your blood sugar is elevated (above a specific target) you should receive insulin to cover that rise in blood sugar. If you are receiving basal insulin (Lantus®, Levemir® or NPH) you should receive that insulin.

Ask your nurse or doctor "what is the plan for my basal insulin dose while I am NPO (not eating)?" If the response is that the medication will be "held" or not given, ask that the "hold basal insulin" order be reviewed. **Your basal dose of insulin may be reduced but SHOULD NOT BE HELD when you are not eating.**

What should I do if more than 30 minutes passes between the time my blood sugar is checked and the nurse arrives with my insulin?

You should question the nurse as to when your blood sugar was checked, the current time and the amount of insulin that he or she is administering to you. If your glucose was checked after your meal, you will need to request that the nurse discuss with the doctor how much insulin you should receive as this is an "after meal" glucose check. Ask that your blood sugar be rechecked so that the dose of insulin is adequate to cover your current blood sugar.

Secondly, you want to convey to the nurse how diligent you are at taking care of your insulin at home and request that your blood sugar be checked when your meal arrives.

How do I know that the insulin being prescribed or administered is the correct dose for me?

It is important to ask the nurse the amount of insulin and the insulin preparation (type) that is being administered to you while in the hospital. You are the expert in your diabetes management, and if the dose does not seem correct, you should seek clarification. Your home dose may be adjusted to help achieve blood sugar control.

May I use my own equipment in the hospital?

If your admission to the hospital is planned, you should discuss this question with your doctor who cares for you and your diabetes. Most hospitals have policies restricting the use of personal equipment in the hospital. However, since hospitals do not have insulin pumps or comparable equipment many will let you self-manage your diabetes using your own insulin pump. Many hospitals will permit you to use your own personal lancets, as they tend to be smaller in size. They may also allow you to use your own personal meter so that you may continue to maintain a record of your blood sugars while you in the hospital.

In the presence of a caregiver, using the "2-drop blood method" you will lance your finger and obtain a drop of blood for your meter and another drop of blood will be obtained for the hospital meter. **However, the blood sugar that will be treated is the blood sugar that was obtained by the hospital meter.** The hospital meter is tested for accuracy and is compared to the blood sugar values obtained by the hospital laboratory.

May I have my family bring in food from home?

If you have concerns about your meals in the hospital, discuss this with your bedside nurse. A consult to the dietitian may be necessary to help you select foods on your menu that you prefer and that meet any dietary restrictions. Bringing in food from home is discouraged because of food safety concerns. There is a potential risk of food that has been contaminated or food that has not been adequately temperature controlled during transport to the hospital.

It is important for your caregivers to be aware of the amount of food that was eaten as well as the nutrient makeup of the food. It is difficult to determine calorie or carbohydrate content from food that has been made at home. This is another reason that bringing in food from home is not advised.

I wear an insulin pump; may I wear it while I am in the hospital?

Discuss this concern with your doctor or surgeon who will be admitting you to the hospital. Determine whether the hospital has a policy permitting patients using an insulin pump to self-manage their diabetes while in the hospital. You may request to see the protocol for insulin pump self-management before you are admitted.

In order for your caregivers to support your efforts to control you blood sugar with your insulin pump, you will need to:

- Tell your nurse of any concerns you have about using your pump safely in the hospital.
- Sign legal documents provided by the hospital that identify your role and your caregiver's role in facilitating the use of your insulin pump.
- Bring all necessary supplies to wear your pump successfully. This includes the pump reservoir, infusion set (insertion device if needed), dressing equipment and extra batteries. The hospital pharmacy will dispense the insulin prescribed by your doctor.
- Provide information about your basal rate(s), insulin to carb ratio and correction factor.
- Remind caregivers that you are receiving insulin through a pump.
- Maintain bedside logs recording your carbohydrate intake and amount of insulin you have bloused (administered) for your meal.
- Change your insertion site a minimum of every three days or if you have two unexplained blood sugars readings in a row greater than 300mg/dL.
- Be agreeable to removing your pump and transitioning to another insulin regimen when you go to the operating room, X-ray, magnetic resonance imaging, cardiac catheterization or if you become too ill to manage your pump safely.

What do I need to know about managing my diabetes safely when I go home?

It is likely that your medication or insulin regimen was modified while you were in the hospital. You want to make sure that you have a good understanding if there is a change that will be made to your home diabetes regimen.

What is DSME?

DSME stands for Diabetes Self-Management Education. It is an outpatient education program that educates patients and their loved ones about managing all aspects of diabetes care. Class topics include:

- Eating healthfully
- Being physically active
- Monitoring blood sugars, and interpreting results
- Taking medications safely
- Reducing risks of complications
- Setting personal goals for managing diabetes

It is important to receive formal education in diabetes management from diabetes experts. DSME classes are taught by nurses, dietitians and pharmacists who have received extensive education in diabetes and care daily for patients who have diabetes.

Over 70% of patients who have diabetes never receive a referral for outpatient diabetes education. A well-informed and educated patient is more successful in managing their diabetes.

If you or your loved one has Medicare, they are covered to receive a total of 10 hours of initial education within a continuous 12-month period and two hours of follow-up education every year after that. One of the hours can be given on a one-to-one basis. A physician's prescription is required and should be provided by your discharging physician or primary care physician.

To be eligible for 2 more hours of follow-up education, you will need another written referral from your doctor.

Before going home, you should be able to answer "YES" to all of the following statements:

✓ I know the names, dosages and directions for taking ALL my medications that have been prescribed.

✓ I have prescription for my medications, insulin, insulin syringes or pen and pen needles and blood sugar testing supplies.

✓ I have a blood glucose meter and know how to use it correctly if I have been instructed to monitor my blood sugars.

✓ I know how often to test my blood sugars.

✓ I know what foods and the amounts of foods I should choose to eat healthfully.

✓ I know the signs of a low blood sugar and how to manage an event correctly.

✓ I know the signs of a high blood sugar.

✓ I know when and whom to call about blood sugar values that are too high or too low and cannot be managed safely at home.

✓ I have received a referral to an outpatient dietitian for medical nutrition therapy (MNT).

✓ I have received a referral to an outpatient Diabetes Self-Management Education (DSME) program.

✓ I have received a referral to a social worker or case manager if I have financial or social concerns that will prevent me from obtaining medications, education or testing supplies to manage my diabetes.

Are there INTERNET resources
where I can learn more about diabetes?

Listed below are sites that contain very helpful information. All of the content contained on these sites have been written by diabetes experts.

Academy of Nutrition and Dietetic
www.eatright.org

American Association of Clinical Endocrinologists
www.aace..org

American Association of Diabetes Educators
www.diabeteseducator.org

American Diabetes Association
www.diabetes.org

American Heart Association
www.heart.org

Diabetes Exercise and Sports Association
www.diabetes-exercise.org

National Diabetes Information Clearinghouse
www.diabetes.niddk.nih.gov

National Institute on Aging
www.nih.gov/nia

The Neuropathy Association
www.neuropathy.org

USDA Center for Nutrition Policy and Promotion
www.cnpp.usda.gov

USDA ChooseMyPlate
www.ChooseMYPlate.gov

Weight-control Information Network
http://win.niddk.nih.gov

Heart Attack (Myocardial Infarction)

Theresa Cary & Deborah Klein

Being rushed to the hospital with a heart attack is frightening. Having crushing chest pain and difficulty breathing is almost an indescribable experience. This chapter will discuss the symptoms of a heart attack and the care that is provided to help you get well.

What is a heart attack?

A heart attack (myocardial infarction) occurs when the blood supply to the heart muscle is blocked. It is often caused by a clot that formed in a one of the blood vessels that bring oxygen to the heart. A heart attack may result in permanent damage to the heart muscle.

What are the symptoms of a heart attack?

Symptoms of a heart attack include:

- Chest pain or discomfort that lasts for more than a few minutes or goes away and comes back
- Pain or discomfort in other areas of the upper body

- Difficulty breathing or shortness of breath
- Sweating or "cold" sweat
- Fullness, indigestion or choking feeling
- Nausea or vomiting
- Light-headedness
- Extreme weakness
- Anxiety
- Rapid or irregular heartbeats

Symptoms of a heart attack are not relieved by rest or oral medications. A heart attack requires emergency medical attention.

Why is it necessary to call 911 if I think I am having a heart attack?

If you think you are having a heart attack, do not attempt to drive yourself to the hospital. You require emergency care provided by trained personnel. The risk of driving yourself to the hospital is that your symptoms could make it difficult to drive safely, you could collapse or pass out, or you could suffer a cardiac arrest while you are driving and injure someone else.

What will the paramedics and emergency medical personnel do when they arrive at my home?

Once emergency help arrives, they will talk to you about your symptoms and begin diagnosis and treatment, which includes electrocardiogram (ECG, EKG) and blood tests. They will administer oxygen and medications and monitor you continuously while in the ambulance. They will also be communicating to the emergency department about your condition.

What will happen when I get to the emergency department?

When you arrive in the emergency department several things will be done very quickly. Your heart rate and rhythm will be evaluated, and your pain will be treated. Once the severity of the heart attack is known, your medical plan will be created. The following tests, procedures and treatments may be utilized:

- Electrocardiogram (ECG, EKG) is a recording of your heart's electrical activity, rhythm and rate. It is printed on graph paper and helps determine the extent of damage to your heart muscle and which part of your heart is affected.
- Blood Tests will be drawn to measure levels of cardiac enzymes, or markers, to see if you have had a heart attack. When your heart muscle cells are injured, enzymes are released into your bloodstream. By measuring the levels of these enzymes, the size of your heart attack and when it occurred can be determined.
- Medication (thrombolytic therapy) can be used to dissolve blood clots in your coronary arteries.

These "clot buster" drugs, if given within a few hours from the time a heart attack begins, can greatly reduce the amount of damage caused to the heart muscle. Cardiac catheterization may or may not be performed.

- **Cardiac catheterization** (also called cardiac cath or coronary angiogram) is a diagnostic procedure in which a long, thin tube is inserted into an artery and guided to the heart. A special dye is injected, and X-ray movies are taken to evaluate or confirm the presence of coronary artery disease, valve disease or disease of the aorta; evaluate heart muscle function; and/or determine the need for further treatment, such as an interventional procedure or surgery. An interventional procedure may be performed to open narrowed coronary arteries to improve blood flow to the heart.
- A **balloon angioplasty** is a procedure in which a small balloon at the tip of the catheter is inserted near the blocked or narrowed area of the coronary artery. When the balloon is inflated, the fatty plaque or blockage is compressed against the artery walls, and the

diameter of the blood vessel is widened to increase blood flow to the heart.

- A **stenting procedure** may be performed in combination with a balloon angioplasty. A stent is a small, metal mesh tube that acts as a scaffold to support the inside of the coronary artery to hold it open. Over several weeks, the artery heals around the stent.

Your doctor may order additional tests, such as an exercise stress test, echocardiogram, or Positron Emission Tomography (PET) scan to evaluate your heart and/or provide additional treatments. These tests may be done while you are in the hospital, or you may have them done after you go home.

Why do I need to go to the intensive care unit (ICU) if I've had a heart attack?

Individuals who have had a heart attack need very close monitoring and observation. You will be given medications that are very potent and can change your physical condition rapidly. Caregivers in the ICU can quickly respond to minute-to-minute changes that a person with a heart attack may experience.

If you have undergone a cardiac catheterization or angioplasty, your nurse will examine your catheter insertion site frequently. It is important to tell the nurse if you notice any bleeding from this area or your leg, foot or hand begins to feel numb or tingle.

How long will I be in the hospital after my heart attack?

You can expect to stay in the hospital two to five days. Your bedside nurse will develop a plan of care and review it with you each day. It's important that you know and understand the plan. This plan will include medications, activity, diet and any tests or procedures that may be scheduled for the day.

Your heart rhythm will be monitored continuously via electrodes connected to a monitor or small box which you may wear. Your blood work and heart rhythm will be evaluated daily to determine how well you are recovering.

It's important to recognize that you are still at risk of having another heart attack. Please notify your nurse right away if you have chest pain or other symptoms similar to what brought you to the hospital. Although your cardiac condition may have been treated, you still have cardiac disease and remain at risk for future heart attacks.

Even though your heart muscle begins to heal soon after a heart attack, the healing process continues for about eight weeks. Just like damaged skin, a scar will form in the damaged area of your heart. This scar tissue cannot function as well as healthy heart muscle, so your heart may not pump as well as it did before your heart attack. How much less work it can do depends on the size and location of the scar. Prompt treatment and restoration of blood flow can keep the extent of heart damage to a minimum.

What can I do to reduce my risk of having another heart attack?

Your bedside nurse will teach you and your loved ones throughout your hospital stay. Treatment of coronary artery disease involves reducing your risk factors, taking medications as prescribed and seeing your doctor for regular visits. Treating coronary artery disease is important to reduce your risk of a stroke or another heart attack

Reducing your risk factors involves making lifestyle changes, including the following:

- Quit smoking.
- Make changes in your diet to reduce your cholesterol. Low-fat, low-sodium and low-cholesterol foods are recommended.
- Control your blood pressure.

- Manage your blood sugar if you have diabetes.
- Limit alcohol to no more than one drink a day.
- Increase your exercise/activity level to help achieve and maintain a healthy weight and reduce stress. Ask your doctor before starting an exercise program, and consider participating in a cardiac rehabilitation program.
- Take medications as prescribed.

Why do I need to take pills for my heart?

Medications that are prescribed all do something different to improve the function of your heart and your overall health. These medications improve your heart function, control your blood pressure, lower your cholesterol and protect against life-threatening heart rhythms. If you are unable to take medications as prescribed, it is important to notify your physician or nurse. An alternative medication may be available.

How do I care for the incision in my groin if I've had a cardiac catheterization?

If you had a cardiac catheterization, there may be a bandage (dressing) over the catheter insertion site (also called the wound site). It is normal for the catheter insertion site to be bruised for several days. The site may also be slightly swollen and pink, and there may be a small lump (about the size of a quarter) at the site. Follow these care instructions:

- Wash the catheter insertion site at least once daily with soap and water. Place soapy water on your hand or washcloth, and gently wash the insertion site; do not rub.
- Keep the area clean and dry when you are not showering.
- Do not use creams, lotions or ointments on the wound site.
- Wear loose clothes and underwear.
- Do not take a bath, tub soak, go in a hot tub/whirlpool, or swim in a pool or lake for one week after the procedure.

- If the site was closed with sutures (stitches), your bedside nurse will tell you how to care for your incision.

What do I need to know about going home after having a heart attack?

Before going home, you should be able to answer "YES" to all of the following statements:

✓ I know the names, dosages and directions for taking ALL my medications that have been prescribed.

✓ I have prescription for my medications.

✓ I have a plan to obtain all of my prescribed medications.

✓ I know what to do if I miss a dose of my medication.

✓ I have a plan to attend cardiac rehabilitation.

✓ I have a follow up appointment with a cardiologist and my primary care provider.

✓ I know which symptoms warrant a call to my primary care provider.

✓ I know how to care for my cardiac catheterization site.

✓ I know when to call 911.

✓ I have received a referral to an outpatient dietitian for Medical Nutrition Therapy (MNT).

✓ I have received a referral to a social worker or case manager if I have financial or social concerns that will prevent me from obtaining medications.

Are there INTERNET resources where I can learn more about heart attacks?

American Heart Association
www.heart.org

National Heart, Lung and Blood Institute
http://www.nhlbi.nih.gov/

Heart Failure in Adults

Nancy M Albert

Heart failure becomes more common as people age. It is the leading reason for hospital admissions for people over the age of 65. It is also a major cause for readmission to the hospital. If you, or a loved one, have a diagnosis of heart failure, there are important lessons to learn so that symptoms and complications can be reduced.

What is heart failure?

Heart failure is a chronic condition without a "cure." It can be managed and controlled by YOU, with help from your loved ones, so that you live a longer and more quality filled life. Some aspects of caring for or controlling your heart failure involve heart failure self-care maintenance and self-care management strategies.

Heart failure is not a disease. Rather, it is a clinical condition that can be caused by many different diseases, such as a heart attack, high blood pressure, diabetes, obesity, smoking, a virus, genetic predisposition, atrial fibrillation (an abnormal heart rhythm commonly found in the elderly), alcohol and drug abuse (especially cocaine) and others.

How is heart failure diagnosed?

Your doctor will ask you questions about your family history and any symptoms you may be having. Your doctor will also listen to your heart for abnormal sounds and listen to your lungs for possible buildup of fluids. Your feet, legs, abdomen and veins in your neck will be checked for signs of swelling.

Diagnostic tests may be performed such as an EKG (a test that shows the rate and rhythm of your heart), a chest X-ray and imaging studies (most often, an echocardiogram) which show the structure or blood flow of your heart may also be performed. Your doctor will want to diagnose heart failure in the early stages so that you can be treated and begin to feel better. The goals of treatment for heart failure are:

- Treating the underlying cause of your heart failure
- Reducing your symptoms
- Preventing your heart failure from getting worse
- Improving the quality of your life
- Teaching you how to manage your heart failure

What are signs and symptoms of heart failure?

Some common signs and symptoms of heart failure include:

- Shortness of breath with activities or at rest
- Fatigue
- Difficulty breathing when lying flat
- Coughing
- Swelling in your ankles, legs or abdomen
- Rapid or racing heartbeat
- If heart failure is advanced, you may have a decrease in appetite or forgetfulness

What are symptoms of worsening heart failure?

The most common signs or symptoms of worsening heart failure include:

- Shortness of breath with activities or even at rest. For example, getting short of breath climbing 1 flight of stairs (13 steps).
- Difficulty sleeping at night without adding extra pillows.
- Waking up at night and needing to sit up in bed to breathe better.
- New or worsening swelling in your feet, ankles, legs, fingers, hands and/or belly (abdomen). You may notice your pants, shoes or socks fit differently or that your belt around your waist is too tight.
- New or worsening fatigue when carrying out activities and walking. Feeling like your legs are tired or you need to take a nap.
- New or worsening coughing at night when lying flat.
- Feeling your heart race or even having chest discomfort when you lay on your left side. This may be due to increased pressure on your heart while lying in this position.
- Sudden or unexplained increase in weight. Generally, a weight gain of 4 or more pounds that occurs in a short period of time (days) and is not explained by a large appetite may be due to worsening heart failure.

What should I know about being hospitalized for heart failure?

A hospitalization for worsening heart failure means your heart function has decreased. A decrease in heart function may be due to simple fluid overload, but more than likely it means your organs cannot handle the work needed to maintain normal function. People who are frequently hospitalized for worsening heart failure tend to have a shorter lifespan.

Our goal is to keep you out of the hospital, as heart failure is a chronic condition that should be treated in an office setting whenever possible. It is important to follow the recommendations of your doctor and nurses, so that your heart function can strengthen and stabilize other body organs.

When stabilized, you have the best chance of feeling good and enjoying life.

When hospitalized for heart failure, your treatments are based on your symptoms, the medical problems that lead to worsening heart failure, your medical history and the ways you have been caring for yourself at home.

A typical hospital length of stay for medically-managed heart failure is 4 to 6 days, but may be fewer days when patients respond quickly to intensive therapies or when the cause of worsening heart failure is not too complicated.

How can I work with my caregiving team when I am in the hospital?

If you have a history of heart failure and are in the hospital, there are 5 actions you should take to ensure the best health possible or to improve your health.

1. Pay attention to your salt intake when you select foods from the hospital menu.

   - Fresh fruits and vegetables are always great choices.
   - Grilled chicken and fish are the best way to eat meat and fish proteins. Breading contains a lot of salt and should be avoided.
   - The "salty 6" that you should stay away from are (1) soups, (2) lunch meat, (3) pizza, (4) fried chicken, (5) bread or rolls, and (6) sandwiches made with bread, lunch meat and high-salt condiments, like ketchup.
   - Other salty foods to avoid include many snacks, like potato chips, pretzels, ham and pickles (or other pickled foods).
   - Avoid sauces (spaghetti or brown sauce) and salad dressings that are high in salt content. One way to eat less, but get the flavor you crave is to ask for the sauce or dressing on the side, so that you control how much you use.

- Ask your nurse to assist you with food choices if you are unsure, or ask to speak with a dietitian.

2. Ask your bedside nurse about your medications. Your nurse should teach you the names of medicines, why they are being used, side effects, the best way to take them, and what to do if you forget a dose after you go home.

    - If you believe that medications you were using at home for heart failure are different than what you are receiving in the hospital, ask your nurse to explain the differences. Medications are an important part of managing heart failure.
    - The more you know about how medications work and what they do and do not do, the better able you will be to take care of yourself properly, after discharge from the hospital.

3. Know your body weight, as it can tell your caregivers if you have too much fluid in your body. If you were not weighed, ASK your nurse to do so every day.

    - Write down your weight, and think about how you are feeling at your current weight. Are you short of breath in bed or when walking in the hallway? Are you less tired than when you came in to the hospital?
    - Compare your weight from when you came into the hospital with today's weight.
    - Ask your doctor or nurse what your "ideal 'dry' weight" is. Dry weight is your weight when your fluid level is normal (no excess fluid is in your blood vessels and tissues).

4. Ask your nurse if you should limit fluid intake. Many adults with heart failure do not need to monitor and watch their fluid intake,

but during a hospital stay for worsening heart failure due to fluid overload, you may be asked to limit your daily fluid intake when in the hospital and even after you go home. Your nurse and nursing assistants will closely monitor how much fluid you eat or drink. If your fluid is restricted, consider the following:

- Use the smallest amount of water possible to swallow medications.
- Suck on hard candy or flavored suckers if you are thirsty (use sugar free if you have diabetes). Eat grapes to get extra moisture in your mouth.
- Avoid milk or milk products, as they will make you thirsty.
- Keep track of your fluid intake. Write it down. Fluids include soups, coffee, soda, popsicles, jello™ and other frozen liquids. If you suck on chopped ice, the amount of 'liquid' you take in is equal to one-half the amount of ice you eat. For example, 1 cup of ice is equal to ½ cup of liquid. Generally, the goal is to take in less than 6-8 cups of fluids per day.

What care will my bedside nurse provide to monitor and treat my heart failure?

During your hospital stay for heart failure, your bedside nurse will:

- Evaluate your blood pressure, heart rate, oxygen level and respirations to be sure your values are normal, or as expected. If not, the nurse will communicate with your doctor or other caregivers.
- Assess how your heart is beating (your heart rhythm). As the heart muscle becomes more abnormal, some people develop abnormal heart rhythms. Sometimes abnormal heart rhythms can threaten life. Your nurse will monitor your heart rhythm and communicate problems to your doctor or other care providers.
- Monitor your fluid status. Your nurse will compare your weight today with your weight yesterday, and may also compare the

amount of fluids you took in with your urine output to see if you are retaining fluids (building up extra fluid) in your blood vessels and tissues.

- Treat new or worsening heart failure symptoms or any new problems.
- Determine how you respond to new and chronic heart failure medications. A hospital admission is an excellent time to "tweak" your medication regimen. Nurses assess how you respond to your medications. If you feel different or experience new problems, it may be caused by a drug's side effect. Please talk to your doctor or nurse immediately if you experience unusual body sensations or symptoms.
- Encourage you to be physically active every day (more than just sitting in a chair; for example, walking in the hallway).
- Assess your knowledge about heart failure and heart failure treatments. Nurses should ask you questions about heart failure topics, so they can learn what education to focus on. Common heart failure topics are: low sodium diet, daily activities and exercise, medication management, daily weight monitoring, signs and symptoms of excess fluid or worsening fatigue, sleep patterns, emotional responses to heart failure and social support.
- Teach you about heart failure (what it means, its chronic nature, consequences and how you can control your symptoms). Your nurse will also tell you what self-care actions to take if your condition worsens.
- Assess your understanding of heart failure and heart failure treatments after delivering education.
- Assess your ability to take care of yourself after discharge and discuss post-discharge care coordination needs with you and your healthcare team.
- Discuss post-discharge care expectations, including a visit with your doctor or nurse within 7 and 30 days of discharge.

Why is being physically active important when a person has heart failure?

Your heart is a muscle, and like all muscles, it needs exercise. Physical activity and exercise help to condition your heart and other muscles so that, over time, you will be able to 'do more' without excess fatigue and shortness of breath. It is normal to become sweaty, have an increase in heart rate and to become short of breath when exercising. These effects will become less common over time, even when you increase your level of activity. Get out of bed each day, and move around your hospital room and in the hallway, unless you are instructed not to do so.

- Stop your activity for 1 minute if you cannot walk and talk at the same time or if your heart rate seems too rapid. If you become dizzy or nauseated with activity, you may be over-exerting yourself. After 1 minute, resume your activity at a slower pace if possible.
- Remember to:

  1. Start slow and increase physical activity and exercise over time.

  2. Exercise to a goal (achieved over time) of 30 minutes of moderate activity (brisk walking) 5 days per week.

- Plan activities for the time of day you have the most energy. Take breaks and mix sit-down activities with physical activities and exercise. Pace yourself!

What are self-care maintenance behaviors that I should be performing to manage my heart failure?

To increase your chances of living a longer life and having a high quality of life, you will most likely need to make changes in your lifestyle (heart failure self-care maintenance behaviors). Your loved ones should assist you with these behaviors:

- Find ways to increase your activity. Make a goal to complete physical activity 5 days a week for 30 minutes each day. You can carry out activity and exercise all at 1 time per day (30 minutes) or in smaller segments; for example, 10 minutes at 3 different time points per day.
- Monitor your body every day for signs and symptoms of new or worsening heart failure, and notify your doctor or nurse of changes.
- Weigh yourself on the same scale every morning, before eating, wearing the same type of clothing, and write it down. If you gain more than 4 pounds from your ideal weight, notify your doctor or nurse.
- Purchase and eat foods that are low in sodium. Your doctors and nurses will provide you with information about restricting your sodium intake. Your recommended sodium intake may be as low as 2,000 mg a day or may be closer to 3,000 mg a day. Read food labels for serving size and mg/sodium per serving. Fresh foods are best.
- Monitor sodium intake when eating out of your home.

Avoid fast food restaurants, as many foods are high in sodium. Avoid pizza, fried chicken, deli sandwiches and soups. Choose salads, vegetables, grilled chicken or fish and fruits.

- Ask the cook NOT to use salt when seasoning or cooking food.
- Avoid foods and drinks known to be high in sodium content.
- Be careful of "heart healthy" choices on menus; they are usually low in fat, but may be high in sodium (salt).

- Review the menu before eating out to be sure there are good food choices for you. Suggest restaurants to family and friends, as needed.
- When going to someone's home, bring your own foods if you know the menu may be high in sodium.
- Avoid alcoholic beverages (beer, wine and hard liquor).

Take heart failure medications as prescribed by your doctor or nurse.

- Do not skip medications if you are feeling fine. Heart failure can get worse "silently."
- If you have side effects from your medications, contact your doctor or nurse.

If you regularly miss taking medication doses, talk to your doctor or nurse. There may be alternative medications that may work better for your lifestyle, or your nurse may be able to help resolve problems.

- See your heart failure doctor regularly. Most people with heart failure should have their condition monitored 1-4 times per year, even when feeling fine.
- Early post-discharge care (within 7 days of discharge) is very important, even if you are feeling fine.
- Most people still have excess fluid in their blood vessels and tissues after hospital discharge. At your first appointment, your doctor or nurse will assess your fluid status carefully and may revise your medication plan based on findings.
- Receive an influenza vaccine every year, unless your doctor has instructed you not to; receive a pneumococcal vaccine every 5+ years, unless your doctor has instructed you not to.

What should I share with my nurse about difficulty following my heart failure plan of care?

Nurses want to deliver personalized care to you, so that you have the best chance of going home and not being re-hospitalized. If you are having trouble with any of the following, ask your nurse to assist you.

- Confusion; forgetfulness
- Inability to take your medications as prescribed
- Lack of transportation for follow up care – trouble keeping doctor's or nurse appointments
- Inability to eat fresh, low-sodium foods due to costs, travel, chef preferences or other living situations
- Feeling depressed or overwhelmed
- Unsure of how to monitor for worsening heart failure
- Problems you have that make walking and physical activity difficult
- Lack of social support

Your bedside nurse can discuss your needs with other members of the healthcare team and enlist their help in identifying resources to help you.

What are heart failure self-care management actions?

Heart failure self-care management actions are taken when you or your loved ones notice worsening of heart failure symptoms. Monitoring yourself daily for worsening condition and taking actions to reverse the problem or stop the problem from getting worse may help you live longer and avoid hospitalization. If you start self-care management actions and your symptoms do NOT improve, contact your heart failure doctor or nurse.

If you notice 2 or more of the following: new or worsening shortness of breath; need to sleep on more pillows, or sleep upright; need to sit upright at night (from a sound sleep) to breathe easily; inability to carry out activities of daily living without stopping and taking breaks; unexpected weight gain of more than 4 pounds; increased night time urination (more urine or more trips to the bathroom) and new or worsening swelling in feet, ankles or abdomen:

1. Decrease fluid intake to less than 8 cups/day for 3 days.
2. Decrease the sodium in your diet to less than 2,400 mg/day for 3 days.
3. If your doctor or nurse allows you to take an "extra" diuretic medication, follow their plan of care. If not, contact your doctor or nurse and ask about taking an extra dose of diuretic. Do NOT take an extra dose of diuretic medication without your doctor or nurse's guidance.
4. If you have not been weighing yourself daily, start now. Weigh yourself every day and record findings. Look for a decrease in weight.
5. If your worsening symptoms do not go away and/or your weight does not decrease by 4 pounds on day number 4 (after 3 days of self-care management), contact your doctor or nurse immediately.
6. If your symptoms and weight improve, schedule an appointment to see your doctor or nurse within 1 month.

If you notice you are more fatigued or taking more or longer naps, or if your heart rate (when at rest) is up by 8+ beats per minute or your blood pressure is lower than previous readings, ensure you are taking your heart failure medications as ordered, and contact your doctor or nurse for an appointment to be seen within 2 weeks.

What do I need to know about managing my heart failure safely at home?

It is likely that your medications were modified while you were in the hospital. You want to make sure that you have a good understanding of any changes to your heart failure regimen.

Before going home, you should be able to answer "YES" to all of the following statements:

✓ I know the names, dosages and directions for taking ALL my medications that have been prescribed.

✓ I have a prescription for any new medications.

✓ I know when and how often I need to weigh myself.

✓ I know what foods, and the amounts of foods I should eat to eat healthy.

✓ I know symptoms I may feel or changes in my body I may see that can be signs of worsening heart failure.

✓ I know when and whom to call about my symptoms that cannot be managed safely at home.

✓ I have received a referral to a social worker or case manager if I have financial or social concerns that will prevent me from obtaining medications or supplies to manage my heart failure.

Are there INTERNET resources where I can learn more about heat failure?

Listed below are sites that contain very helpful information. All of the content contained on these sites has been written by heart failure experts.

Academy of Nutrition and Dietetics
www.eatright.org

American Association of Heart Failure Nurses
http://aahfnpatienteducation.com/

American College of Sports Medicine
www.acsm.org

American Council on Exercise
www.acefitness.org

American Heart Association
www.americanheart.org

American Psychological Association
http://locator.apa.org

Centers for Disease Control and Prevention, Patient Education
http://www.cdc.gov/heartdisease/materials_for_patients.htm

Heart Failure Society of America
www.HFSA.org

Kidney Disease

Lynda Newman & Julie Simon

Hospitalizations are frequent for patients with chronic kidney disease (CKD) and those patients with end stage renal disease (ESRD) who require dialysis. If you or a loved one has kidney disease, you may be fatigued, frustrated and discouraged with the daily activities associated with managing your disease.

Whether you are admitted for your kidney disease or other illness, you want to make certain that your caregivers are knowledgeable about your self-management practices or dialysis regimen. Never be reluctant to remind your caregivers that you have chronic kidney disease.

What should I tell my nurse and other caregivers about how I manage my kidney disease at home?

- The most challenging thing about living with your kidney disease. Sharing this concern with your caregivers can increase their awareness of your personal needs.
- Medications you are taking and how are you actually taking them.

- Changes you may have made to the amount or frequency of your medications. Please tell your doctors and nurses if you are not taking prescribed medications, if you are forgetting to take your medications or if you are taking less than the prescribed amount.
- The medications you are not taking because of unpleasant side effects.
- Financial concerns that are preventing you from taking the medications you are prescribed.
- Your dry/target weight.
- If you do not have a working scale at home.
- The reasons why you may not have been able to go to dialysis or perform your home dialysis.
- Ideas about why you are having trouble with your fluid balance.
- The supports you have at home, including people to assist you and emotionally care for you.
- The transportation arrangements to healthcare appointments or dialysis.

How might things be different in the hospital than what I'm used to at home?

You may be given medications or undergo procedures that your kidney specialists have told you may be harmful to your kidneys. However, there are times during a hospitalization where the need to investigate your problem outweighs the risk of doing the procedure or taking the medications. Careful consideration will be used by your doctors and nurses when these procedures or medications are necessary for further diagnosis and your recovery. Your doctors and nurses will explain each test to you before it is performed. If you do not understand the reason for the test, be sure to speak up and receive answers to your questions that reassure you.

Dialysis, including peritoneal dialysis, may be done at different times than your usual time when you are at home. Dialysis may be done for a longer or shorter length of time, depending on your needs.

What should I expect from the nurses who take care of me?

Nurses are a great source of wisdom and knowledge in helping you cope with your kidney disease as well as helping you in the daily management of your disease. They will pay close attention to your weight, fluid intake and output, and your appetite.

Your nurses will closely monitor your weight to be sure you are not gaining too much weight in extra fluid. Weights are usually taken early each morning. If no one weighs you, be sure to remind the nurse before you eat your breakfast. Weights taken while standing up are much more accurate than when taken lying in a bed.

Your nurse will evaluate the balance of what you take in (intake) and what you eliminate (output). This helps your caregiving team to assess whether your kidney function is worsening or improving. Nurses need to know everything that you drink (intake), and everything you lose (output) by urine, vomit or diarrhea. You will be given containers for collecting your output. Be sure you do not flush anything without putting on your call light for the nurse or aide so it can be measured.

Your nurse can answer your questions about nutrition as well as consult a dietician. Your nurse will inspect your dialysis fistula, catheter or graft, if you have one in place. He or she may also provide you with information about caring for your dialysis fistula, catheter or graft.

How do I participate in having my needs met during my hospital stay?

Ask questions about any new medications, treatments or concerns you have about caring for yourself at home. If you do not understand something your doctor has told you, SPEAKUP and ask for a different explanation. Keep a note pad by your bed, and write down your questions as they come to you, so you don't forget. Never be afraid to ask a question.

Request your caregivers wash their hands. You can expect caregivers to either wash their hands or use foam hand sanitizer before and after they provide care to you. They should also clean their hands again before touching your dialysis line access.

Many patients with end stage renal disease will require placement of a fistula or graft for dialysis. Fistulas and grafts are surgically-created areas, often in the arm, that are used for hemodialysis. If you know you will be getting a fistula or graft in the future, declare your dominant arm "off limits" to any IVs or blood draws as much as is possible. If that arm must be used, ask that the nurse or lab technician use the smallest needle and draw blood from your hand or as close to your hand as possible. Avoid having blood drawn from the vein located in the bend of your arm.

If you have a fistula or graft, you know that blood pressures and intravenous lines or blood draws should not be performed in or on that arm. Check your fistula or graft for the thrill (the "buzzy" feeling) four times a day. A good way to remember this is to check it at each meal and bedtime. If you are unsure of how to do this, ask your nurse to teach you.

If you have a line for dialysis access, dialysis nurses and technicians are the only caregivers who should be using the line. It should not be routinely used for antibiotics and infusions outside of dialysis.

Tell your nurse right away if:

- You notice any redness, pain, bleeding or swelling in your fistula, graft or line.
- You are experiencing more shortness of breath, fatigue or swelling in your feet, ankles or legs.
- The thrill on your fistula or graft feels less strong.

What do I do if I feel I need more or different care than is being provided?

Never be afraid to ask why, if you notice that your caregiving team is doing things differently than how you were taught to manage your kidney disease at home. Asking can act as a gentle reminder for your caregivers. Being in the hospital can provide you and your loved ones with opportunities to refresh your learning or update your knowledge. Expressing your concern and asking questions will help you and your caregivers be on the same path.

The person who knows you best is YOU. Tell your caregivers what works for you. Hospital routines and activities (sleep, meals, etc.) can sometimes be adjusted to more closely match what you do at home to manage your kidney disease. Keeping things more familiar is often helpful for your healing process.

If you would like your loved ones or significant others involved in your care, tell your bedside nurse. The involvement of family or friends can make discharge easier.

How do I know if my kidney function is getting worse?

Here are some common symptoms of worsening kidney function:

- Being very tired
- Feeling cold all of the time
- Tightness in shoes and rings

- Puffy face
- Difficulty breathing
- Changes in taste
  - metal taste in the mouth
  - meat makes you nauseated (if it did not use to)
  - breath smells like ammonia
- Feeling nauseated all the time
- "Fuzzy" thinking
- Urine is dark and you make less than you used to
- Constant itching

If you are experiencing any of these symptoms, you should call your nephrologist's (kidney doctor's) office.

What are the stages of Chronic Kidney Disease (CKD)?

There are five stages of Chronic Kidney Disease. Each stage is described by specific symptoms and laboratory values. Your nephrologist will ask you to have blood drawn to test your Glomerular Filtration Rate (GFR). The GFR is the rate at which the kidneys filter waste. GFR is one useful measurement of your kidney function.

- Stage 1: signs of mild kidney disease, greater than 90% of kidney function remaining
- Stage 2: signs of mild kidney disease with reduced GFR, 60-89% of kidney function remaining
- Stage 3: Signs of more serious kidney disease, 40-59% of kidney function remaining
- Stage 4: Signs of severe kidney disease, 15-29% of kidney function remaining
- Stage 5: Signs of end stage renal failure, less than 15% of kidney function remaining.

Dialysis is usually required when the disease reaches Stage 4 and 15-29% of kidney function remains.

How will I know what I can and cannot eat?

If you have Stage III Chronic Kidney Disease, you should work on making your diet "Heart Healthy." That means trying to keep your intake of salt (sodium) to fewer than 2,000 mg per day. Many foods contain several types of fat. Some are better for you than others. Choose foods that are low in saturated fats, cholesterol and trans fats. A diet high in saturated fat, cholesterol and trans fats can add extra strain to your heart and the blood vessels that supply blood to your kidneys. Choose lean meats, low fat cheeses and lots of vegetables and fruits. Ask to speak with a dietitian. You can also look for ideas on www.choosemyplate.gov.

Dieticians are experts in healthy eating and can provide valuable information to help you create a menu that incorporates your dietary restrictions. If you have Stage IV or V Chronic Kidney Disease or are on dialysis, you **need** to work with a dietitian. Along with the heart-healthy choices, you may need to restrict foods that are high in potassium and phosphorus. This can feel odd because many of the foods on this restricted foods list are healthy foods – but only for people whose kidneys work.

What can I do to manage bothersome symptoms caused by my kidney disease?

People with CKD often battle constipation. This is made worse if you are on pain medications for any reason. Working with a dietitian can help to make certain that you get the most fiber and fluids in your diet that you are allowed. Let your nurse know if having regular bowel movements is a problem for you. A stool softener may be added to your medication routine.

People with CKD often suffer from dry itchy skin. This is due to higher levels of phosphorus, blood urea nitrogen (BUN) and creatinine in your bloodstream. Limit showers or baths to less than 10 minutes. Apply moisturizer to still damp skin. Camphorated lotions (example: Sarna TM) can help with itching.

What do I need to know about managing my condition safely at home?

Before going home, you should be able to answer "YES" to all of the following statements:

✓ I know when to call 911.

✓ I know the names, dosages and directions for taking ALL my medications that have been prescribed.

✓ I have prescriptions for my medications.

✓ I have a plan to obtain all of my prescribed medications.

✓ I know what to do if I miss a dose of my medication.

✓ I know when my next dialysis session is scheduled.

✓ I know how to care for my dialysis access (fistula, catheter).

✓ I have an appointment with my nephrologist.

✓ I know when I am scheduled to have blood work performed.

✓ I know my dry/target weight.

✓ I know which symptoms warrant a call to my primary care provider.

✓ I have received a referral to a social worker or case manager if I have financial or social concerns that will prevent me from obtaining medications.

Are there INTERNET resources where I can learn more about kidney disease?

American Association of Kidney Patients
www.aakp.org

Kidney Trust
www.kidneytrust.org

National Kidney Foundation
www.kidney.org

National Kidney and Urologic Diseases Information Clearinghouse
kidney.niddk.nih.gov

Renal Support Network
www.rsnhope.org

Liver Disease

Anita White & Shannon Rives

Your liver has an important role in keeping the body running properly. The liver is responsible for many important functions in digestion, blood clotting and breaking down chemicals and medications. Because of all of the important activities your liver performs, it is affected by prescription medications, diet, alcohol and over-the-counter (OTC) medications.

Are there many kinds of liver disorders?

Because the liver is involved in so many important activities, there are a number of disorders that can begin in the liver and have an effect on the rest of the body:

Hepatitis – This is caused by a virus which results in swelling of the liver. Hepatitis can also be caused by non-infectious factors such as obesity, excessive drinking and drugs. There are vaccines to prevent against Hepatitis **A and B, but not C, D and E.**

Cirrhosis- This is permanent damage to the liver that has occurred over time. The liver cells become scarred and are unable to function correctly.

Liver Cancer – It begins in the cells of your liver and is known as hepatocellular carcinoma. There are other kinds of liver cancers, but they are quite rare.

Liver Failure – There are many causes of liver failure, including infections, genetic diseases and excessive drinking over time.

Hemochromatosis - This condition allows iron to be deposited in the liver, which results in damage to the liver.

Primary sclerosing cholangitis – This is a very rare disease and the cause is unknown. This disorder causes inflammation and scarring of the liver.

What kinds of symptoms require an admission to the hospital?

Patients with liver disorders are usually admitted to the hospital because of changes in their mental status (difficulty thinking or making sense), shortness of breath, extra fluid around the abdomen or bleeding.

How can I participate in my care?

It is important to remain open and honest with your caregivers. When you are admitted to the hospital, you may be asked many questions. Your answers help your caregiving team to create a plan for your care. Please be sure to share information or express your concerns about any of the following:

- Use of drugs, alcohol, over-the-counter (OTC) medication or herbal supplements
- Increased pain or discomfort in the abdomen
- Trouble sleeping at night or feeling too sleepy
- Forgetfulness
- Irritability
- Bleeding

- Shortness of breath

How will my liver condition affect my body?

Symptoms of liver disease can be vague. If you have known chronic liver disease (CLD) you need to be aware of the symptoms. Liver disease can cause the body to go through many physical changes. The goal of living with liver disease is to achieve a balance of wellness and symptom management. The functions of the liver support other body systems. So when the liver is sick you can see the effects in different parts of the body (for example, the skin). Your body may not look the same as you remember. You may even have moments when you don't act the same or feel like yourself. Below is a list of common body changes and other words that you may hear them called by your doctor or nurse.

- **Ascites** (a large belly): Ascites happens when fluid accumulates in your abdomen because the liver is leaking fluid into the abdomen. Large amounts of fluid can result in shortness of breath and difficulty walking.
- **Jaundice** (yellow skin): Jaundice is seen when the body is not able to filter toxins. The yellow color comes from a yellow pigment called bilirubin.
- **Petechiae** (red spots on the skin): Petechiae are caused by small blood vessels bleeding under your skin. Disorders of the liver can make it hard for blood to clot.
- **Encephalopathy** (confusion): Encephalopathy is caused by toxins building up in your body and affecting your brain.

What will my caregiving team do to help manage my symptoms?

Treatment for your liver disorder will begin while you are in the hospital and continue after you are discharged. Your caregiving team will order a diet that is low in salt to help your body get rid of extra fluid. You may also begin to take a diuretic, or water pill, to get rid of extra fluid.

You will be given medications to rid your body of the toxins that can sometimes impair your thinking and ability to move around easily. These medications may cause you to have loose stools and to move your bowels more frequently. Let your nurse know if your bottom becomes sore from using the toilet or bedpan.

Your nurse or nursing assistant will keep a record of all the times you urinate or move your bowels. This information is important and helps your nurse and healthcare team determine how well the medication is working.

Some of the treatments may make you feel weak. If you do feel weak, let your nurse know so that special attention can be provided to prevent you from falling and offering assistance with meals.

What do I need to know about managing my condition safely at home?

Keep taking all of your medicines as prescribed, even if you feel better. Your caregiving team may ask you to have your blood drawn frequently. Remember to keep appointments for blood tests. This is one way that your doctor can monitor your recovery.

Keep a healthy lifestyle! Watch your weight, and eat fresh foods from all food groups. Try to increase intake of high fiber foods. Abstain from alcohol and smoking.

Before going home, you should be able to answer "YES" to all of the following statements:

✓ I know the names, dosages and directions for taking ALL my medications that have been prescribed.
✓ I have prescriptions for all of medications.
✓ I know how many bowel movements I can expect to have during a 24-hour period and what to do if I have more or less.

✓ I know what foods and the amounts of foods I should eat to eat healthfully.

✓ I know which over the counter medications I should avoid or take in limited amounts (ex: acetaminophen or acetaminophen-containing products).

✓ I know the symptoms that require a call to my caregiving team. These symptoms include increased shortness of breath (SOB), increased abdominal girth, bleeding from the rectum, coughing up blood and confusion.

✓ I know who to call if my condition worsens or if I have a concern.

✓ I have received a referral to a dietitian to assist in the selection of healthy foods.

✓ I have received a referral to a social worker or case manager if I have financial or social concerns that will prevent me from obtaining medications or other home supplies.

✓ I have received information about Alcoholic Anonymous or Narcotics Anonymous if appropriate.

Are there INTERNET resources where I can learn more about liver disease?

Academy of Nutrition and Dietetics
www.eatright.org

Alcoholics Anonymous
www.aa.org

American Association for the Study of Liver Diseases
http://www.aasld.org

American Liver Foundation
http://www.liverfoundation.org

Centers for Disease Control (CDC)
www.cdc.gov

Chronic Liver Disease Foundation
http://www.chronicliverdisease.org/

Hepatitis B Foundation
www.hepb.org

Hepatitis C Support Project
http://www.hcvadvocate.org/

Multiple Sclerosis

Marie Namey & Catherine Skowronsky

ultiple sclerosis (MS) is a disease in which your immune system attacks the protective sheath (myelin) that covers your nerves or the nerves themselves. This damage disrupts communication between your brain, spinal cord and the rest of your body. There's no cure for multiple sclerosis. However, there are medications and therapies to help speed recovery from attacks, modify the disease activity and treat the symptoms. An individual who has multiple sclerosis may be admitted to the hospital for treatment of an infection, an adjustment in medication or to treat a complication related to immobility.

What can I expect from my nurse when I am in the hospital?

Your nurse will likely spend more time with you than any other healthcare provider. It's important to share with them how you are, whether you are newly diagnosed or have been admitted with a disease flare. Your nurse can provide you with education and information to help manage your condition.

Your nurse will work with other members of your caregiving team; they will be your advocates and support system.

What information should I share with my caregivers about my multiple sclerosis when I am admitted to the hospital?

You and your loved ones are the experts in your experience with multiple sclerosis. In fact, you may have managed some very severe symptoms of your multiple sclerosis in your home in the past. Your caregiving team will ask many questions to assure that your care routine is not unnecessarily interrupted during your hospitalization. Please share with your caregiving team the following information:

- A list of the medications you are currently taking.
- Information about how you take your medications at home. This should include the time of day, which medications are taken together and any other special information related to your medications.
- Your own plan for handling missed or late doses of medications.
- Whether you receive an immune modifier. If you self-inject or receive an intravenous dose of an immune modifier, tell your caregiving team when you received the last dose and when the next dose is due. Please remember to share any information about how you pre-medicate for doses of an immune modifier to reduce side effects.
- How you manage exacerbations at home and how long they usually last.
- How much assistance you usually need with bathing and dressing. Your need for assistance may change when you are experiencing an exacerbation.
- How much assistance you usually need with getting up or moving around. Please bring any assistive devices you use with you to the hospital. Your loved ones may take them home if the hospital is able to provide a suitable substitute for you to use during your stay.

How will my medications be managed when I am in the hospital?

Your medication regimen will best be determined by the reason you were admitted to the hospital. It is possible that you were admitted for adjustments to medications used to treat your multiple sclerosis or for side effects related to those medications. If that is the case you may expect some changes to your medication routine. You may always ask for a list of your medications and the times at which they are scheduled. Your caregiving team will let you know their plans for adjusting medications used to treat your multiple sclerosis.

If you were admitted to treat an infection or complication of immobility, there will be some medications added to your regimen. Your caregiving team will let you know if they expect that you will need to receive antibiotics or other therapies after you are discharged from the hospital.

How will my loved ones be involved with my care while I am in the hospital?

Chances are you have a team of loved ones or individuals at home who help you manage your disease and remain active in your activities of daily living. Your loved ones are welcome to participate in your care while you are in the hospital if they wish.

Your loved one may also wish to be present at your bedside when the physician or team of physicians caring for you visits daily. This is a good time to have questions answered and to learn the plan of care for the rest of your hospital stay.

Loved ones provide care and support for individuals facing a chronic illness when they devote time to their own health and wellness. Your hospitalization may offer a time for your loved one to rest and replenish so they may remain available to you after your hospitalization.

What should I do to avoid a fall while I'm in the hospital?

Multiple sclerosis produces a wide range of symptoms, including weakness, spasticity and loss of balance. These symptoms may result in impaired mobility and increase your risk of falling.

Your bedside nursing team frequently assesses your risk for falling while you are in the hospital. Infection or other illness in addition to multiple sclerosis can increase your risk even more than what is normal for you. Based on your level of risk, the nurses will develop a plan of care with your participation to help keep you safe. It is important that you understand and participate in the plan.

The plan is designed to prevent you from falling while you are in the hospital. Your bedside nurse may ask you not to get out of bed without calling for help. He or she will also discuss with you and your loved ones the precautions that are needed to keep you safe from falling when you are in the hospital.

Please refer to the chapter titled Preventing Falls for further information.

What do I need to know to manage my condition at home?

Planning for discharge starts the moment that you are admitted to the hospital. Your caregiving team will discuss their plan of care with you and work with you to discuss your progress daily.

There are several things you can do to minimize complications related to your multiple sclerosis once you are discharged:

Follow-up with your healthcare team as directed.

- Take your medications as prescribed.
- Eat a well-balanced diet.
- Maintain a healthy weight.

- Develop an exercise routine. (You may need the help of a physical therapist.)
- Get adequate rest.
- Stop smoking.
- Learn techniques for stress management.
- Accept the help of family and friends.

Before going home, you should be able to answer YES to all of the following questions:

✓ I know the names, dosages and instructions for taking all of my medicines.

✓ I have prescriptions for the medications I will be taking.

✓ I have a follow-up appointment with my neurologist.

✓ I know whom to call if my condition worsens or if I have a concern.

✓ If I am continuing intravenous treatment at home, I have plans in place for home care or my loved ones have been instructed on how to safely administer the medications.

✓ I am aware of strategies to prevent falling at home, work and in public

✓ I know how to promote my own personal safety by modifying my home environment.

Are there INTERNET resources where I can learn more about multiple sclerosis?

National Multiple Sclerosis Society
http://www.nationalmssociety.org

Multiple Sclerosis Association of America
http://mymssa.org

National Institute of Neurological Disorders and Stroke
http://www.ninds.nih.gov/index.htm

Parkinson's Disease

Kate Klein

P arkinson's disease can make being in the hospital more challenging. The most common causes for patients with Parkinson's to be admitted to the hospital include changes in balance and walking, falls, difficulty swallowing and/or choking, and changes in mood or memory. This chapter will describe how your caregivers will work with you while you are in the hospital.

What do I need to tell my caregivers about how I am living with Parkinson's disease when I am admitted?

Provide the name and phone number of your Parkinson's disease neurologist to your caregiving team.

Let the staff know if you have a deep brain stimulation (DBS) implant. Bring the access review or magnet device to turn the stimulator on and off for procedures. This is important information to share with your caregivers because the deep brain stimulation implant can send signals that affect other medical equipment.

If you are enrolled in a research study, provide information explaining the experimental drugs, and phone the study coordinator to let them know you are in the hospital.

How will my medications be managed while I am in the hospital?

Be sure to bring an accurate list of your current medications, their dosages and the times that you take them. Include all over-the-counter medications and supplements. Your nurse will provide the list of medications and dosages that have been ordered by your doctor. If any medication that you routinely take for your Parkinson's disease is not ordered by your doctor, please tell your nurse. If your medication is abruptly or unexpectedly stopped, you may be at risk for developing a severe reaction called neuroleptic malignant syndrome. Symptoms of neuroleptic malignant syndrome include extreme rigidity or stiffness, high fever and confusion. Do not take your own medication from home unless you have discussed this with your doctor and nurse. If you are temporarily unable to take your medications by mouth, they may be available as an injection or a patch.

What should I do to avoid a fall while I'm in the hospital?

Your bedside nurse will ask you about how well you move at home and what assistive equipment you use. Your bedside nurse will also ask you about how easily you become tired and how you conserve energy when moving around. Your nurses will create a plan of care with your participation to help keep you safe from falling. You are an important participant in this plan.

Your nurse will have discussed the precautions that are needed to keep you safe from falling with you and your loved ones. The most important safety precaution is not to get out of bed by yourself. Most falls in the hospital occur on the way to the bathroom or in the bathroom.

Sometimes patients with Parkinson's disease have a drop in blood pressure when they change position or stand up. This can cause dizziness or the feeling of being lightheaded. This is another reason why you should call for assistance or call for help when getting out of bed.

It is especially important that you partner with your nursing staff for help to the bathroom. This point cannot be overemphasized as you may feel strong enough to get out of bed by yourself or with a family member but this is strongly discouraged. Please ask for help.

Why is it important to get out of bed or be mobile while I'm in the hospital?

Staying as active as possible is important for all of your body systems, especially your muscles and joints. It also helps in digestion and prevention of complications, such as breathing problems and blood clots.

If a nurse or nursing assistant does not offer to walk with you, ask for help to get up. If you need extra assistance or cannot get out of bed, a physical therapist or occupational therapist may visit to assess your needs and create an exercise plan.

How will I get assistance with eating?

Meal trays are delivered to your room. You should put your call light on if you need help with opening cartons and packages. Make sure that you are sitting up. It is strongly encouraged to eat your meals sitting in a chair.

A speech therapist may visit you to help with your swallowing and speech. There are swallowing techniques that can help you swallow more safely.

A dietitian may visit you to discuss food preferences and food consistency. Several medications that are used to treat Parkinson's disease must be taken before a meal or on an empty stomach. The dietitian will work with your physician, nurse and pharmacist to customize your medication schedule.

What should I do if I notice my loved one becoming confused while in the hospital?

The hospital environment is unfamiliar and can be noisy and disruptive to sleep. Lack of rest and a change in environment may cause delirium in hospitalized patients. Delirium is a sudden change in mental status or confusion that develops over hours to days. Delirium is different than dementia, which is a disease that gets worse over time. Signs and symptoms of delirium include anxiety, restlessness, rapid changes in emotion and hallucinations.

Checking in with your loved one about the day of the week and current events, getting exposure to natural light, avoiding daytime naps and spending time with those who are familiar can help someone with Parkinson's disease reduce confusion or delirium.

Alert your loved one's bedside nurse if you noticed that he or she has suddenly become confused or has had a change in behavior.

Before going home, you should be able to answer YES to all of the following questions:

✓ I know the names, dosages, side effects and directions for taking ALL my medications that have been prescribed.

✓ I know why this (these) medication (s) were prescribed for me.

✓ I know what actions to take it I miss a dose of my medication.

✓ I know how to get this medication refilled.

✓I know how long I need to take this medication.

✓ I know the restrictions to be followed when taking this medications (such as diet, exercise, bleeding risk, intimacy, driving, operating heavy equipment, etc.).

✓ I know how I am going to pay for this medication.

✓ I know how to store this medication at home so that it is not damaged.

✓ I know which foods affect the way my medication works.

✓ I know how alcohol affects the way my medication works.

✓ I know what over-the-counter medications will worsen Parkinson's symptoms or cognitive function.

✓ I know not to take any more or less than the prescribed dose.

✓ I know when and whom to call if I am having a major side effect from my medication.

✓ I know who is going to help me take my medications at home if I need assistance.

✓ I know how to use the equipment that is needed to administer my medication (inhalers, syringes, patches, pumps, etc.).

✓ I have an established routine to take my medications as prescribed.

✓ I know the name and phone number of my Parkinson disease neurologist.

✓ I know the make and model of my deep brain stimulator (DBS), if applicable. I know how to turn the device on and off or instruct somebody on how to turn the device on and off. I have the access review or magnet device to turn the stimulator on and off for future procedures.

✓ I know how to minimize aspiration/choking risk.

✓ I know what precautions to take in my home to prevent falling.

✓ I know who I can call and where I can go if I need management of my symptoms.

Are there INTERNET resources
where I can learn more about Parkinson's disease?

National Parkinson® Foundation
www.parkinson.org

National Institute of Neurological Disorders and Stroke
www.ninds.nih.gov

American Academy of Neurology
www.aan.com

American Parkinson's Disease Association
www.apdaparkinson.org

Parkinson's Disease Foundation
www.pdf.org

Michael J. Fox Foundation for Parkinson's Research
www.michaeljfox.org

Worldwide Education and Awareness for Movement Disorders
www.wemove.org

Parkinson's Action Network
www.parkinsonsaction.org

Surviving Adversity: living with Parkinson's
http://www.survivingadversity.com

Respiratory Disorders

Christina Canfield

If you can't breathe, nothing else matters. Being admitted to the hospital for a breathing problem can be a frightening experience. If you are hospitalized for a respiratory disorder your caregiving team will work with you to ease your symptoms and improve your breathing. This chapter will describe the hospital routine and interventions/treatments that may occur during your hospital stay.

What can I expect from my nurse while I'm in the hospital?

Your nurses will likely spend more time with you than any other healthcare professional. It is important to share information with your nurse. Whether you have been newly diagnosed with lung disease or you have been admitted because your disease has gotten worse, your nurse can provide you with education and information to manage your condition.

Your nurses will perform frequent assessments of your breathing. They will listen to your lungs with a stethoscope several times a day. You may be asked to wear a device called a pulse oximeter on your finger. The pulse oximeter provides a reading of the amount of oxygen in your blood. The pulse oximeter may stay in place 24 hours a day, or it may be placed on your finger as needed.

Your nurse will be at your side throughout your hospitalization to work with you and the other members of the healthcare team. Your nurse is your advocate and support system.

Is there anything I can do when I feel short of breath?

You may feel short of breath for many reasons. Your nurse will work with your healthcare team to create and deliver treatments designed to ease your discomfort. Let your nurse know if it becomes more difficult to breathe. He or she may be able to give you medication or contact the respiratory thera-pist to administer a breathing treatment.

You may feel more comfortable if you sit upright in bed. The hospital bed can be adjusted to help you do this more easily. Sit as high as you can, and take slow breaths through your nose. Exhale slowly out your mouth, counting to 4 as you do so. Some patients find that leaning forward with their elbows on a table is also helpful.

Can I use the same inhaler I use at home?

Your physician will prescribe or "order" inhalers for you while you are in the hospital. While medications, including inhalers, are usually not stored in a patient's rooms, it may be possible for you to keep a short acting "res-cue" inhaler at your bedside. Let your nurse know if you use this inhaler so he or she may keep an accurate record of the medications you have taken.

I feel claustrophobic when I wear an oxygen mask. Is there anything I can do to make it more comfortable?

There are many different ways to give oxygen to hospitalized patients. Each device provides oxygen in a different way. Your caregivers may decide that you need an amount of oxygen that can only be given by a mask that covers your face and nose. The mask needs to fit snugly to give you the oxygen you need. Some patients find that having a fan blow toward their face helps with feelings of claustrophobia and makes them more comfortable.

The oxygen dries out my nose. Is there anything I can use to make it more comfortable?

Oxygen can be drying and irritating to your nose, especially if you are not used to using it. A humidification bottle adds moisture to the oxygen before it reaches your nose. Ask your nurse or respiratory therapist if it is possible to use humidification. It can be helpful to apply a water-based lubricant to the inside of your nostrils. This reduces the dryness and discomfort. Your nurse can provide you with water-based lubricant and show you how to apply it.

How will I know if I need to go home on oxygen?

Your caregiving team may decide you need to wear oxygen at home. Oxygen is prescribed like a medication and should be treated like any other medication. Before you are discharged a respiratory therapist may perform a test called a desaturation study. This is done by placing a device on your finger called a pulse oximeter. The pulse oximeter measures how much oxygen is being carried by your blood. The respiratory therapist may ask you to walk beside him or her or perform some activity. During this time, he or she will monitor your oxygen and watch your breathing. If you have difficulty breathing or getting oxygen to your body, you may need oxygen at home.

Smoking and oxygen do not go together, and there is no safe way to smoke while you are on oxygen. Talk to your nurse, respiratory therapist or oxygen provider about oxygen safety.

What happens if I need to be put on a breathing machine?

Doctors carefully review and evaluate all available information before deciding to put patients on a breathing machine. The main job of our lungs is to inhale oxygen to nourish the body and to exhale carbon dioxide that forms as the body uses oxygen. There are many reasons a patient might need help with their breathing. These include: easing the work that is needed to breathe, helping the body receive and use oxygen more effectively and eliminating carbon dioxide. In many cases breathing machines, also called ventilators, are used for patients who cannot breathe for themselves.

Some patients can receive help with their breathing through a snug-fitting mask connected to a ventilator. This is called Bi-Pap. Others need more support and must have a small air tube inserted through the mouth and into the trachea or wind pipe. Before the tube is placed, your nurse will give you medication that will make you feel sleepy and relaxed. You should not remember the procedure when you wake up.

There are times when the caregiving team decides that it is best to keep a patient "sedated" or in a light sleep while they are on the ventilator. If you are sedated, your nurse will perform frequent assessments to assure you are as comfortable as possible. If you are not sedated, it is important to remember not to pull at or try to remove the breathing tube. It is natural for this tube to feel strange in your mouth and throat. Your nurse and respiratory therapist will help you feel more comfortable by cleaning and moisturizing your mouth and moving the tube from side to side.

Your nurse or respiratory therapist will need to suction your air tube several times each day. Suctioning removes secretions (mucus) to help you breath better. A much smaller tube (suction catheter) is passed through the air tube and secretions are removed. While suctioning is not painful, it can cause feelings of breathlessness. Suctioning is very brief so the feeling of breathlessness will only last a short time.

You will not be able to speak while you are on the ventilator. Your nurse will provide you with paper on which to write or a pre-made letter board so you can point and spell. Many times the letter boards also have commonly used words such as "pain," "cold" and "bathroom" spelled out.

For many patients, the need to be on a ventilator is temporary. Your care-givers will perform assessments to determine whether you are ready to breathe on your own. If it is determined that you are ready to breathe on your own, the tube will be removed and you will receive oxygen from a mask. Your breathing and oxygen will be monitored closely after the tube is removed. It is normal to have a sore throat and hoarse voice for a few days.

If you cannot breathe on your own after a long period of time, the health-care team may ask you or your family if they can place a tracheostomy tube in your neck. A tracheostomy is a surgical opening created in the front of your neck and into your windpipe (trachea). A tube is then inserted into the opening. A tracheostomy tube helps with breathing and can increase your comfort on the ventilator. The tube is not always permanent and may be removed when you are able to breathe on your own.

How do I communicate my wishes for treatment?

It is important that you share your wishes with your family in case you are unable to speak for yourself. It is recommended that you complete an advance directive and a healthcare power of attorney form and provide copies to your loved ones and the hospital any time you are admitted. It is never too early in your disease to get this important task done. Advance directives will let your family and caregivers know what kind of treatments you wish to receive should you become unable to speak for yourself. If you wish to complete these forms while you are in the hospital, tell your nurse and he or she will contact the social work department to assist you with these important forms.

There may come a time when you start to feel like you no longer wish to receive aggressive treatment for your lung disease. Please share this right away with your healthcare providers, including your nurse. There are many things that can be done to keep you comfortable and ease feelings of breathlessness. A palliative medicine team may be asked to work alongside your caregivers to plan your care. Palliative medicine is focused on ensuring comfort and relieving symptoms associated with advanced disease.

What can I do to stay well after I am discharged?

Living with a respiratory disease means making some lifestyle changes you may not have planned. You are probably aware that cigarette smoke can cause respiratory disease and also make it worse. If you smoke, please create a plan to stop. Your nurse can give you more information about the steps to take to stop smoking. If you live with a smoker, please encourage him or her to quit. If your family member is unable to quit, be sure that he or she does not smoke around you or in the areas where you will spend most of your time. Avoiding cigarette smoke will not cure a chronic disease like emphysema, chronic bronchitis or asthma, but it will help you manage your symptoms better and keep you well longer.

People who have been diagnosed with a respiratory disease are more likely to catch illnesses, such as the flu or pneumonia. Both of these common conditions may be prevented by receiving a vaccination. If you've never had a yearly flu shot, get one next flu season. The flu shot does not give you the flu or cause the flu. Most patients experience minimal side effects; such as arm tenderness where the vaccination was injected. If you've never received the pneumonia vaccine, request one before leaving the hospital.

The importance of good hand washing in the prevention of illness cannot be over-stressed. You've seen your caregivers wash their hands or use a hand sanitizer before and after providing care. Follow their example when you are discharged. Wash your hands with soap and water, or use an alcohol-based hand sanitizer after coughing, sneezing or blowing your nose. Wash your hands with soap and water after using the bathroom and before each meal. Wash your hands more frequently if you or a loved one is sick.

Before going home, you should be able to answer "YES" to all of the following statements:

I know the names, dosages and directions for taking ALL my medications that have been prescribed.

✓ I have prescriptions for all of my pills and inhalers.

✓ I have a peak flow meter.

✓ I know how often to monitor my peak flow and what to do if it is out of range.

✓ I know what foods and the amounts of foods I should eat to promote good health.

✓ I know the signs and symptoms of a respiratory infection.

✓ I know when to follow up with my doctor.

✓ I have received a referral for pulmonary rehabilitation (if appropriate) and know how to schedule an appointment.

✓ I know who to call if my condition worsens or if I have a concern.

✓ I have received a referral to a social worker or case manager if I have financial or social concerns that will prevent me from obtaining medications, oxygen or other home supplies.

Are there INTERNET resources where I can learn more about lung disease?

American Lung Association
www.lung.org

Centers for Disease Control and Prevention
www.CDC.gov

The Global Initiative for Chronic Obstructive Lung Disease
www.goldcopd.com

Smokefree.gov (smoking cessation)
http://smokefree.gov/

Seizure Disorders

Erica Yates

Seizures can happen suddenly and sometimes without warning. Many things can lead to seizures, such as epilepsy, low blood sugar, medications and alterations in electrolytes. There are also many different types of seizures that can look very different from each other. For example, during one type of seizure a person may be confused, during another seizure a person may be aware of what is going on but unable to talk and during yet another seizure a person may have full body shaking. Some people will be unaware that a seizure occurred, while other people will know that they have had a seizure.

Because seizures can occur without warning, many people who have experienced seizures will have anxiety about when another seizure will occur. People who have fallen or experienced injuries during their seizure may also have anxiety or be fearful. It is good to share your feelings about seizures with your nurse so that he or she will know how best to assist you.

It is also important that you discuss your seizures with your nurse. Your nurse will want to know what type of seizures you experienced, when your last seizure occurred, how often your seizures occur, how long your seizures last and if you have ever experienced falls or injury with your seizures. Some patients become confused after a seizure occurs. Let your nurse know if you become confused after a seizure. All of this information will help your nurse to plan your care with you to make sure that your goals of care are met.

What will nurses do to keep me safe in the hospital?

One of your nurses' goals is to keep you safe during your hospitalization. Some types of seizures can cause falls and/or injury. Because seizures can be unpredictable, safety measures will be put into place to protect you while you are in the hospital. The side rails on the bed will be padded, and when you are in bed all four of the rails may be in the up position. Equipment such as suction and oxygen may be at the bedside. Suction will be used to clear any vomit or mucous from your mouth. Oxygen may be given to help your breathing.

Even if your seizures are well controlled at home, you are more likely to have a seizure during hospitalization for several reasons. If a dose of your seizure medication is given late or missed for any reason, you will be more likely to have a seizure. The stress of hospitalization may also increase your risk for seizures. Disruption of your sleep may occur during your hospitalization. This may also play a role in increased seizure activity.

What should I do if I feel like I am going to have a seizure?

If you feel that you may have a seizure, you should call the nurse or yell for help. If your seizures happen suddenly and you are not able to call for help before the seizure, please call for assistance once you are able to do so. Your nurse will want to know if you had a seizure so that she can assess your vital signs and neurological status. It is important for the nurse to monitor you for multiple seizures occurring in a short period of time or seizures that last a long time. Nurses and other staff members will come in your room to assist you if a seizure occurs. This may be overwhelming, but they are there to assist you and make sure that you are safe.

Why do I need to call for assistance if I want to get out of bed?

Experiencing seizures puts you at greater risk for falling. You may be asked to call for assistance whenever you get out of bed, including when you get up to go to the bathroom. Not being able to get out of bed on your own may be difficult for you, but the nurses would like to assist you to prevent you from falling or being injured.

How can I expect my seizure medication to be managed while I am in the hospital?

Seizure medications may control, but do not cure seizures. This means that the medications can prevent you from having a seizure if you maintain a steady level of the medication in your body. This is why it is important to make sure your nurse knows that you take seizure medication as soon as you get to the hospital so that you do not miss a dose. If you do miss a dose of your medication, tell your nurse so that you can receive your medication as soon as possible.

It is important to take your medications on time as prescribed. If you miss a dose of your medication the level of the medication in your body will go down and you will be more likely to have a seizure. Missing several doses of your medication may lead to seizures that are different than what you usually experience.

Before going home, you should be able to answer "YES" to all of the following statements:

✓ I know the names, dosages and directions for taking ALL my medications that have been prescribed.

✓ I have prescription for my medications.

✓ I know what changes should be made to my living environment to assure my safety at home.

✓ I know what symptoms require a call to my physician.

✓ I have received a referral to a social worker or case manager if I have financial or social concerns that will prevent me from obtaining medications.

Are there INTERNET resources where I can learn more about seizures?

American Epilepsy Society

https://www.aesnet.org/

Centers for Disease Control and Prevention

www.cdc.gov

Epilepsy Foundation

www.epilepsy.com

International League Against Epilepsy

www.ilae.org

Stroke

Stacey Claus & Amy Young

When your loved one suffers a stroke, it happens suddenly, without warning and its effects can be long-lasting and even life-altering at times. Changes in your loved one's appearance and abilities will vary depending upon the type of stroke and what part of the brain has been affected.

Symptoms of a stroke may include:

- Inability to move arm and/or leg on affected side.
- Inability to move the hand, arm, face, leg like before.
- An area of the body does not feel or have feeling like it did before.
- Words are not clear and might be slurred. Speech may sound thick like your loved one is talking with their mouth full.
- Speaking the wrong words or the inability to get words to come out.
- Drooling from one side of the mouth, or choking on saliva or other liquids.
- Blurred vision, double vision, darkness or complete loss of vision.
- Mood swings, depression, lack of interest in typical activities.

Why is it important to call 911 right away after noticing symptoms of a stroke?

Surviving a stroke and managing its long- term effects can be hard work, but there are many caregivers who are there to help your loved one on the path to recovering. Throughout this hospital admission, your loved one's bedside nurse is the link to putting all the pieces together. Your loved one's nurse will be at the bedside watching their response to questions and strength tests, evaluating their response to ordered treatments, communicating with the medical team, providing a healing environment and educating you and your loved one.

Loved ones are an invaluable resource as an extra set of eyes and ears. You know your loved one better than anyone. When you notice any changes in your loved one, bring it to the nursing staff's attention. It just might be one of the most important pieces of information that they have in determining how well your loved one is doing.

Are there different types of strokes?

There are two different types of stroke: hemorrhagic and ischemic. A hemorrhagic stroke is often referred to as a "bleed" or bleeding in the brain. This type of stroke is caused by a blood vessel that breaks as a result of high blood pressure. Hemorrhagic stroke is not as common, but is the more life-threatening type of stroke. Patients who have had a hemorrhagic stroke tend to be sicker.

An ischemic stroke is often referred to as a "clot" or blockage in the blood vessel. This type of stroke is caused by a blockage in the vessels that supply the brain. This can happen at night while sleeping or during activity. If this type of stroke happens at night, you will notice the changes when you wake up in the morning. Ischemic stroke is the most common type of stroke.

What type of hospital is best for somebody who is having a stroke?

When stroke symptoms are noticed call 911; do not drive your loved one to the emergency room. When 911 is called, your loved one will be transported to a stroke-certified hospital. Primary and comprehensive stroke centers are certified by The Joint Commission which is a national organization that regulates hospitals, to provide high-quality stroke care according to established guidelines. These centers closely monitor patients who have had a stroke and their outcomes to ensure that the best care is being provided. These hospitals are ready to quickly care for and manage your loved one's stroke.

What happens when my loved one arrives at the hospital?

Once your loved one arrives at the hospital, you may feel overwhelmed. You may be asked to describe your loved one's symptoms and when they began. People will be moving quickly asking you or your loved one a lot of questions. They will also ask your loved to do several different things such as:

- Answer specific questions. (For example: What year is it? Who is the President?)
- Show muscle strength by grasping a caregiver's hand.
- Perform specific tasks, such as lifting their arms into the air or sticking out their tongue.

These behaviors provide the team of caregivers with information about the location of the stroke and how it has affected your loved one. The severity of your loved one's stroke will direct the nursing care they need.

Often an intravenous line (IV), which is a thin straw-like tube inserted into a vein, is used to allow medications to be given quickly. A tube may be placed in the bladder. Vital signs, such as blood pressure, pulse (heart rate) and breathing, will be checked very frequently.

What types of tests will be performed on my loved one?

Brain scans are tests that are used to diagnose the type and location of your loved one's stroke. They include the following:

- **Computed Tomography** (CT scan) is a quick diagnostic study that provides pictures of the inside the brain. Patients lie on a table and move into a tube-like machine that takes pictures of their brain.
- **Magnetic Resonance Imaging** (MRI) is similar to a CT scan, but provides more detailed pictures of the brain. Please let us know if your loved one has difficulty laying still or has a fear of small places, also known as claustrophobia.

Your loved one will be moved quickly from the emergency department to radiology (X-ray). It is important to find out if they are experiencing a stroke and if so, which type in order to care for them correctly.

The reason things move very quickly for patients with stroke symptoms is that treatments work best when they are started early. There are cut-off times for being able to treat stroke patients. The "last known well" (LKW) is a very important question that you may be asked many, many times: When is the last time your loved one had no symptoms?

If your loved one has had a stroke, how they are treated depends on many factors. First, is the time since they were last normal (the "last known well" time when they had no symptoms). Second is the kind of stroke (hemorrhagic or ischemic, clot or bleed). Depending on this information, your loved one may be given a thrombolytic (clot busting medication) through the IV or they may be given coagulants or reversal medicine to stop bleeding. They may also be taken to interventional radiology (IR), a special X-ray room where medical staff can do procedures, or to the operating room.

Any of these treatments need to be done quickly to have the best results. The fact that there are many people working very fast does not mean that your loved one is unstable or in danger. Some patients may not need immediate treatment, but will be monitored.

How will I know how my loved one is doing?

Patients who are suspected of having a stroke are continuously monitored for changes in thinking and movement. It may become frustrating to you or your loved one because certain questions and tests will be repeated over and over, sometimes as frequently as every 15 minutes.

Sometimes, stroke may affect a person's ability to breathe normally. If your loved one is unable to breathe, doctors may decide to place a breathing tube through the mouth and into the lungs. This can be uncomfortable, but may only be temporary. The tube will be hooked up to a machine, or ventilator, to help with breathing. Often suctioning of the airway is needed. Suctioning entails using a tube to suck any fluid out of the breathing tube, or mouth, similar to what the dentist uses. This can be uncomfortable. Suctioning by the nurse or respiratory therapist will remove mucus, which will help in breathing.

Lab tests will be drawn to monitor your loved ones' blood counts. Blood sugar may also be performed because the stress of the stroke may cause a rise in blood sugar.

What can I do to prevent complications from my stroke?

There are some well-known complications that occur as a result of a stroke. Two frequent complications are aspiration and blood clots in your loved one's legs.

Aspiration occurs when food, saliva, liquids or medications accidentally enter the lungs. Aspiration happens because either the stroke has affected your ability to swallow or the stroke has made you too sleepy or weak to swallow safely. Aspiration can lead to the development of pneumonia, which will keep you in the hospital longer.

To ensure the safety of your loved one:

- Please refrain from feeding your loved one until the nurse or doctor has given you permission. A swallow screen will be completed by a nurse before anything is given by mouth. It is very important that you are aware when swallowing is a problem.
- Ask the caregiving team for the results of the swallow screen. You will be informed of whether a speech therapy evaluation is needed or if there have been any dietary or feeding recommendations.
- Encourage your loved one to sit upright in bed or in a chair when they are eating, just like at home. If getting out of bed is not possible, then make sure your loved one is sitting upright while taking anything by mouth.
- If it is determined that swallowing is not safe, a small temporary tube may be placed through the nose and into the stomach. This is called an enteral feeding tube, or a nasogastric (NG) tube. The placement of the NG will be checked by X-ray before anything is administered through it.

Venous Thromboembolism (VTE) is commonly referred to as a blood clot in the arms or legs. These can be life-threatening if the clot travels to the lungs.

To help in the prevention of a blood clot:

- Ensure that your loved one is wearing special stockings provided by the hospital called intermittent pneumatic compression (IPC) stockings on both of their legs around the clock. These stockings intermittently squeeze and help keep blood flowing in the legs. The noise and sensation can be bothersome; however, these stockings are an important treatment in preventing blood clots. If your loved is not wearing them when you visit, please ask the nurse.

- Encourage your loved one to get out of bed and move around, even if it starts out slowly. Do not try and get your loved one out of bed by yourself. It is important to call for assistance since your loved one's balance and strength can be affected by the stroke. Physical therapists and occupational therapists are experts in helping patients with strokes begin to recover.

- Become familiar with the medications your loved one is now receiving. Blood thinners are important medications in preventing VTEs. These may be given as injections at first and then as a pill. These shots are usually given in the abdomen and can cause a burning sensation when injected. This is normal and even though it may cause discomfort, the medication is highly effective at preventing the formation of blood clots.

What are the signs that a stroke is getting worse?

Alert your loved one's caregivers if you notice any of the following signs or symptoms:

- Change in ability to communicate
- Increased weakness
- Increased facial droop (crooked face)
- Sudden sharp, throbbing headache
- Inability to pay attention or stay awake

What do I need to know about my loved one's care before leaving the hospital?

During your loved one's hospital stay, the caregiving team will talk to you about many things. Please ask questions, even if the caregivers have answered them before. There is a lot of information. If it is unclear, ask. If you need more information, ask.

Caregivers may ask a lot of questions about home. They are not being nosy. Your loved one's level of function (how well he or she can independently care for themselves) and your home environment may determine where he or she goes when they leave the hospital. If your loved one cannot walk steps and lives in a two-story home, he or she may need to go for further therapy before going home. Your loved one may go home, go to a skilled facility for further treatment or have an order for home care (a healthcare member comes to your home).

Before going home, you should be able to answer "YES" to all of the following statements:

✓ I can name the type of stroke my loved one experienced.

✓ I can identify the risk factors of my loved one having a repeated stroke.

✓ I know when and how to call 911.

✓ I know the names, dosages and directions for taking ALL medications that have been prescribed for my loved one.

✓ I know what to do if my loved one misses a dose of medication.

✓ I have a plan to obtain the prescribed medications if financial concerns exist.

✓ I know the name and contact information of the neurologist who will be caring for my loved one when they leave the hospital.

✓ I know how to assist my loved one to move about safely.

✓ I have the adaptive equipment necessary for mobility (ex: walker, cane, tub grips, shower chair, etc.).

✓ I know what changes in my home environment are needed.

✓ I know how to communicate with my loved and understand his or her needs.

✓ I know what foods and the amounts of foods that can be eaten safely.

✓I know how to administer tube feedings safely.

✓ I know how to problem-solve the tube feeding pump if problems occur.

✓ I know when and whom to call about any worsening condition.

✓ I have a copy of the advance directive or other important paperwork (living will, healthcare power of attorney).

Are there INTERNET resources where I can learn more about stroke?

Centers for Disease Control and Prevention
http://www.cdc.gov/stroke/

The American Heart Association
www.heart.org

The National Stroke Association
www.stroke.org

Vascular Disorders

Kathleen Singleton

This chapter will give you general tips on what to expect, what questions to ask your nurse and what questions you may be asked during your hospital stay. While you are in the hospital the registered nurse and members of your caregiving team will work with you to care for your blood vessel disorder. They will teach you how to care for yourself after leaving the hospital.

Caring for your blood vessel or vascular disorder is a life-long process. This chapter will provide a general overview about care in the hospital and information about blood vessel disorders. Specific questions related to the management of your disease or condition should be directed to your physician or other caregiver professional.

How can blood vessel disorders affect my health?

Disorders of the blood vessel system affect your lifestyle before and after a hospital stay. The blood vessel system is like a two-lane highway. Your blood vessel system has two kinds of one-way lanes: arteries (outgoing lanes) and veins (incoming lanes). Arteries are thicker and pump oxygenated blood from your heart to the rest of your entire body with each heartbeat. Veins are thinner, have valves or flaps and push deoxygenated blood back to your heart. Your treatment plan will depend on which lane of the highway, or blood vessel, is affected. The nurse and healthcare team will guide your care.

By the time a blood vessel disorder brings you to the hospital, it is likely the disease has been going on in your body for many years. Disorders of arteries are chronic; they do not go away and need to be managed for the rest of your life. Disorders of veins may be chronic, and any blood clot in a vein is something you need to tell your caregiving team every time you are cared for. Treatment of arteries and veins is aimed at managing the disorder to allow you to feel better and have the best level of function. Depending on the extent, type or blood vessels involved, you may need to have tests, surgery or take medications. Your length of stay in the hospital depends on your treatment plan and your body's responses to the plan.

There are larger arteries and veins deep in the body. The farther from the heart, the smaller the blood vessel is in size. The blood vessels of the legs, arms, neck and below the stomach are the ones most commonly affected. Surgery can help get rid of clots, bypass blockages, repair a vessel that has ballooned out or open up a narrowed blood vessel. It is important to remember that surgery only fixes a blood vessel crisis. Although a blood vessel may be fixed, the blood vessel disorder is not cured; it requires continued care by you, your nurse and the healthcare team. Untreated blood vessel disorders can lead to heart attack, stroke, amputation or even death.

Everybody is on the blood vessel highway of life. Men over 50 years and women who have gone through menopause are at risk for blood vessel disease. A family history of high blood pressure, altered cholesterol levels or blood vessel disease puts you on the express lane for blood vessel disorders. Sometimes there are few, occasional or no warning signs or symptoms of a blood vessel disorder, until the disorder is well under way. These are things no one can change.

Conditions such as high blood pressure, diabetes, altered cholesterol levels, heart disease, stroke, kidney failure needing dialysis, getting older and obesity stress the entire blood vessel system. Other risk factors that affect blood vessels include: smoking, lack of physical activity, cold temperatures, using tools or machinery that vibrate, injury to muscles or ligaments, infection or emotional stressors. Some of these risks can be managed and changed. It is important that you talk with your healthcare team about lifestyle changes you can make to reduce these risks as much as possible.

The nurse will teach you about survival skills that help you manage your blood vessel disorder. Three things you and your nurse can work to achieve are managing the pain, signs and symptoms of a blood vessel disorder; keeping you active or mobile; and learning about healthy life choices.

Why is it a problem when arteries do not work correctly?

Arteries transport blood from your heart to the body. The blood contains oxygen and other nutrients that are important for your tissues, organs and cells to function properly. In arterial blood vessel disorders, the flow of oxygenated blood to the most distant body parts is restricted. Body parts farthest from the heart, like your fingers and toes, are at the greatest danger when blood flow is blocked or slowed. However, organs such as your kidneys, brain and intestines may also be affected.

Normally blood flows through arteries at a steady pace matching your heartbeat. This gives you pulses that can be felt in your neck, arms, legs and feet. Being able to find, feel or hear the strength of pulses tells the nurse and caregiving team a lot about the blood flow within your arteries. Your pulses may be checked many times a day and even at night. The nurse will need to check your pulses by touch or with a listening device called a Doppler. Sometimes pulses are hard to find even with the Doppler. The nurse may ask you to lay still so that the pulse can be located. The nurse may put an

"X" with a pen or marker over the spot where the pulse is the strongest. It is important for the "X" to remain even after your daily bath or shower.

Why is it a problem when veins do not work correctly?

Remember that veins carry blood back to your heart. Blood vessel disorders of veins are usually the result of the valves or flaps in the veins losing their ability to open and close. Blood is not able to easily move along.

Blood clots can form when the flow of blood slows or stops. Although a blood clot can be life-threatening, it can be managed with medications. Anticoagulant medications (blood thinners) such as Coumadin®, Lovenox® or heparin keep your body from making new clots. Some anticoagulants require you to have blood tests to follow your blood levels closely. Some anticoagulants can be taken by mouth while others must be injected daily.

You may need to wear compression stockings every day for several months because the stockings provide support to your blood vessels and help with circulation. It is important that you remove the stocking once a day and look at your legs for any new redness or sores. The stockings should be snug and the right size.

When blood flow in veins is slowed or stopped, your arm or leg will swell, hurt and may even leak straw-colored fluid. Your legs may feel tight, tired or heavy. Your pulses are not altered. You may have more pain at the end of the day. Your lower legs may become darker in color or hardened. Sores or ulcers may develop above the ankle on the inner part of your lower leg. There are several treatments and types of ace wraps or stockings that can be used to heal the sores or ulcers. Even when healed, these sores or ulcers may come back.

How can I work with my caregiving team while I am in the hospital?

If you have vascular disease and are admitted to the hospital, your caregiving team will be interested in pain, mobility and appearance of your limbs. The answers you can provide for these questions will help the team create a plan that best meets your physical and emotional needs.

- Do you have pain, discomfort or fatigue in your legs or feet when walking?
- Do you feel achiness, burning or cramping of your legs or feet when walking or with exertion?
- Does the achiness, burning or cramping of your legs or feet lessen when you rest?
- Do you have aching, burning or fatigue in your feet or toes at rest?
- Do your legs hurt when they are raised above your heart?
- Do you have any callouses, sores or wounds on your lower legs, feet or toes?
- Do you have any sores that do not heal?
- Have you had any toes or parts of your foot removed? If so why?
- Do you wake up at night and then sit in a chair or recliner with your feet hanging down?
- When do you have the most pain – in the morning, during the day or at night?
- How has your life changed because of your arterial or venous disorder?
- Have you noticed any swelling or discolorations in your legs or feet?
- Have you noticed less hair or loss of hair on your legs or feet?
- Have you noticed thinning of your skin, shininess or pale color of your legs and feet?
- Have you noticed any changes in your toenails – thickening, unable to see the nail bed or loss of toenail(s)?
- Do your arms or legs turn reddish-blue in color?

- Do your toes turn blue when you hang your feet down?
- Are any parts of your toes black, brown and leathery?
  Has anyone ever told you that you have weak pulses or they were unable to find a pulse in your legs or feet?

What do I need to know about going home to manage my blood vessel disorder?

The following recommendations will help you live well in and out of the hospital:

✓ Ask questions.

✓ Manage pain.

✓ Get adequate exercise.

✓ Take medications properly.

✓ Manage your diabetes.

✓ Keep your blood pressure under control.

✓ Stop smoking.

✓ Manage life and occupational stressors.

✓ Manage your weight.

✓ Bond with your nurse and the healthcare team.

Before going home, you should be able to answer "YES" to all of the following statements:

✓ I know the modifications that need to be made to my home while I am recuperating.

✓ I know the names, dosages and directions for taking ALL my medications that have been prescribed.

✓ I have a prescription for any new medications.

✓ I know who can help me recover at home.

✓ I can identify resources and stress-management techniques to help with help me cope with my blood vessel disorder.

✓ I know how to inject my blood thinner if I am going home on an injectable medication.

✓ I know what foods to eat and what foods to avoid if I am taking a blood thinner.

✓ I know when I can resume driving.

✓ I know what symptoms require a call to my healthcare provider.

✓ I know the restrictions on my activity (walking, climbing stairs, exercise, etc.).

Are there INTERNET resources where I can learn more about blood vessel disease?

American Heart Association
www.heart.org

Amputee Coalition
http://www.amputee-coalition.org/

Centers for Disease Control and Prevention
www.cdc.gov

National Heart, Lung and Blood Institute
http://www.nhlbi.nih.gov/health

Vascular Disease Foundation
http://vasculardisease.org/

Part Four:

Partnering with Your Caregivers when You Require Surgery

"One of the greatest diseases is to be nobody to somebody"
Mother Teresa of Calcutta

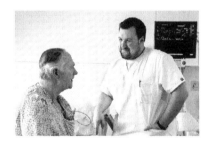
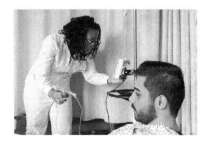
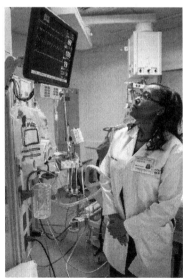

Bariatric Surgery

Karen Schulz

B ariatric surgery is a journey. By the time most patients arrive at their surgery day, they have been through months of evaluation and preparation and are looking forward to the physical transformation the surgery will provide. Your active role in the immediate days after your surgery may mean the difference between going home on time versus staying an additional day. This chapter will describe your postoperative care in the hospital.

What Can I Expect When I Wake Up from Surgery?

As you wake up from surgery, you may feel some discomfort over the abdominal area. Your bedside nurse will monitor your vital signs and pain level. It is important to let your nurse know how you are tolerating your pain and to request pain medication BEFORE you become too uncomfortable. You may have a pain pump which you will control by pushing a button to dispense medication into your intravenous line (IV) when you need it. The pain pump has a maximum rate and will not give you more than is safe.

You will not be permitted to drink fluids, but may ask your nurse if you are permitted to have ice chips or something to rinse out your mouth.

Why do I need to get out of bed on the day I have surgery?

You will be asked to get up and take a walk or two on this day. Your bedside nurse or nursing assistant will be with you to support you as you walk for the first several times. Walking is one of the most important things you can do to improve circulation, prevent blood clots, increase deep breathing and encourage your digestive system to "wake up" after surgery. The anesthesia given for surgery often slows down digestion, and walking will encourage your intestines and stomach to return to normal function.

How will my pain be controlled?

Your surgeon will choose the best method to relieve your pain after surgery. Your caregivers will frequently ask you about your pain level. Pain management is different for each patient, so it is important to express your pain level so that it can addressed.

Simple measures such as using a pillow for splinting your abdomen, changing your position or walking can help reduce pain. Many patients find music soothing. It may be to your benefit to bring along CDs or a MP3 player with your favorite playlist.

Will eating right after surgery be a problem since my stomach will be so small?

You will be on a "bariatric clear liquid" diet for the hospital stay. This diet includes things like broth, gelatin and sugar-free beverages and will be specifically measured as to not overwhelm your stomach pouch. When you are home, you will begin the full liquid diet, which includes the protein shake.

Some patients require an X-ray after surgery to make sure that the pouch is functioning. The test requires you to drink sips of a contrast fluid to observe how liquids pass through your stomach. Once the results are received, your nurse will let you know when you can begin sipping clear liquids. When you have been cleared to drink clear liquids, sip very slowly from a small medicine cup. Do not use a straw.

Why do I have to wear special stockings?

When you are in bed you should be wearing stockings that pump to enhance the circulation in your legs. These socks are commonly called "intermittent pneumatic compression stockings." They help prevent blood clots by applying and releasing pressure on your legs. When getting back into bed, please ask your nurse to reapply the stockings. Some patients report that the stockings are hot or uncomfortable; however, it is necessary to wear them to prevent complications.

How will I feel when I get home?

You have spent months, possibly years, preparing yourself for this surgery. It is not uncommon to have mood swings after surgery or to question your decision for surgery when you are in the early post-surgery days. Discomfort, food aversion and the fact you have not yet lost weight makes it a challenging time, and now that surgery is complete patients often feel a sense of loss or regret. Please know this is normal and these feelings will pass. A few weeks after surgery, most patients experience control over food and a good deal of weight loss, which makes it all worth the hard work of the surgery experience.

Prepare yourself for a couple challenging weeks at home. Know that sipping fluids, including your protein drink, is a full-time job in the beginning. As the surgical swelling decreases and your diet increases, eating and drinking will get easier. Please continue to follow the diet that your surgeon and dietitian discussed with you before your surgery.

How long will I need to stay in the hospital?

That depends upon the type of surgery you have. Patients who have undergone laparoscopic sleeve gastrectomy typically spend 1 to 2 days in the hospital. Those who had laparoscopic gastric bypass spend approximately two days in the hospital. Patients who had duodenal switch or revisional bariatric surgery may require an additional day or two, depending on their individual progress.

What do I need to do to take care of my wound at home?

Stitches are placed just beneath the surface of your incisions. These stitches do not need to be removed. They will be absorbed by your body in about 6 weeks. Occasionally, you will find a small white string at your incision site. This is not a problem. Your surgeon will trim this piece of string at your next visit.

Many patients will have a bulb drain that encourages fluid around the area of your pouch to leave the body easily. This drain may be removed before you leave the hospital, or your surgeon may have you care for it at home for one week. Your nurse will teach you how to empty the drain at home and measure the fluid output. Drain removal just takes a few seconds. Most patients report drain removal to be an unusual pulling feeling, but not painful.

Look at your incision every day to check for signs of infection. Call your surgeon if you notice any of the following:

- An increase in pain or pressure around the incision
- More redness or swelling
- Pus-like or foul-smelling drainage
- Area is warm to touch
- Fever, chills or fatigue

Wear loose clothes that won't rub on your incision. You may wear a dry dressing over the incision to prevent clothing from rubbing. The skin around your incisions may feel numb. This usually goes away over time.

May I shower after surgery?

You may shower daily with soap and water to cleanse your incision.

- Do not rub vigorously over your incisions; simply let water run over your incision to rinse.
- Pat the area dry with a clean dry towel.
- Do not use lotions, powders or salves on your incision
- Avoid tub bathing, swimming or using a hot tub until your incisions have healed and your surgeon has approved you to do so.

How can I manage my pain at home?

You will be given prescriptions for pain medication. If you prefer not to take prescription medication, check with your physician. You may be able take Tylenol® instead of the prescribed pain medicine, but do not take both at the same time.

It is not unusual to have some shoulder pain after surgery. Walking is the best way to relieve this discomfort. A heating pad on your shoulder blades or the upper abdomen may also provide relief. This pain should gradually subside over several days.

How will my tastes and food preferences change after surgery?

Your stomach needs time to heal before solid foods are introduced into your diet. It is very important to follow the diet progression exactly. You may have some distaste for foods that were previously tolerable or pleasurable. These taste changes are normal and should return to normal in the weeks and months to follow. Your dietitian has provided you with the information you will need to manage your meals after surgery.

What kind of activity am I permitted to do at home?

It is common to feel weak and tired right after surgery. Your body is recovering from the stress of a major operation. Rest when you feel tired.

- Increase your activity slowly. Take a walk at least 2 to 3 times per day. Gradually increase the distance you walk each day.
- Do not stay in one position for more than one hour while you are awake.
- You may climb stairs, but you may need some help at first. Make sure someone is with you the first time.
- Do not do any strenuous exercise such as jogging, tennis or weight lifting until approved by your surgeon at your first check-up appointment.
- Do not pull or push heavy objects for the first two weeks after surgery.
- Do not drive until your surgeon clears you to do so. You must be off of all narcotic medications before you begin driving.

When recovering at home, what over-the-counter medications can I take?

Vitamin Supplements are very important and need to be taken for the rest of your life. Refer to the supplement guidelines in your diet packet for specific instructions.

- You **MAY** take the following over-the-counter medicine:
- Adult quick dissolve or liquid Tylenol® for headache or mild incision discomfort.
- Thera-Flu®, Dimetapp®or Triaminic® elixirs for cold symptoms.
- Kaopectate for loose stools.
- If you are having more than 6 watery stools per day for more than a week after surgery, please call your physician's office.

- If you are tolerating solid foods, have not had a bowel movement and you are feeling constipated, you may try an over-the-counter stool softener such as Colace® or docusate sodium.
- If the stool softener does not work, try Phillips Milk of Magnesia®.

You **MAY NOT** take Non-steroidal anti-inflammatory medications as they will irritate your stomach. These medications include: Motrin®, Aleve®, ibuprofen, Naprosyn®, Advil®, Vioxx®, Daypro®, Celebrex®, Bextra®, Lodine®, Toradol®, aspirin, Pepto-Bismol® and Alka-Seltzer®. If you are unsure about the use of a medication, ask your pharmacist.

When should I begin weighing myself?

During your hospital stay, it is common to gain 15 to 20 pounds. This is due to the fluids given to you around the time of surgery that stay with you for a few days. We recommend that you do not weigh yourself until at least 5 days after surgery, when the fluid has mobilized and left your body.

What symptoms require a call to my surgeon or a trip to the emergency department?

If you experience any of the following symptoms, please contact the Bariatric Surgery Program right away or go to the emergency room immediately.

- A temperature higher than 101.5 F
- A heart rate of greater than 120 beats per minute (or more than 20 beats in 10 seconds)
- Shortness of breath that does not improve with 5 to 10 minutes of rest
- New chest pain or shoulder pain
- One arm or leg appears noticeably larger than the other
- Calf pain
- Black or bloody stool
- Vomiting blood

- Persistent nausea, vomiting or dry heaves
- Cloudy, dark and/or foul smelling urine
- Your incision(s) open up, become red, swollen, tender or have new drainage
- Abdominal pain that is not relieved by your pain medication
- Painful, frequent urination or inability to urinate

What do I need to know to be safe at home?

Before going home, you should be able to answer "YES" to all of the following statements:

✓ I know the names, dosages and directions for taking ALL of my medications that have been prescribed.

✓ I have prescriptions for all of my pills.

✓ I know what foods and the amounts of foods I should eat.

✓ I know the signs and symptoms of an infection near the area where I had surgery.

✓ I know which activities are encouraged and permitted until I visit my surgeon.

✓ I know when to follow up with my surgeon.

✓ I know who to call if my condition worsens or if I have a concern.

Are there INTERNET resources where I can learn more about bariatric surgery?

American Society for Metabolic and Bariatric Surgery
https://asmbs.org/

Medline Plus Topics: Weight Loss Surgery
http://www.nlm.nih.gov/medlineplus/

Cardiovascular Surgery

Myra Cook, Kelly Haight & Marian Soat

The news that you or a loved one needs open heart surgery is frightening. This news can come as a shock or may have been anticipated if you have been experiencing increasing or worsening chest pain, irregular heartbeats or shortness of breath. Recovering from surgery is hard work, but with the expertise of your caregiving team and the love and support of your family and friends, your recovery will progress as expected.

Patients who receive open heart surgery recover in the Intensive Care Unit (ICU). After 1 to 3 days in the ICU, patients are usually moved to a different area, which is sometimes called a "step-down" unit. Think of your stay in the intensive care unit as the time needed to stabilize after such significant surgery, and the step-down-unit stay as the time spent preparing your body and mind for going home.

What can I expect while I am in the ICU?

While you are in the ICU you will notice that your nurse spends a lot of time at your bedside. This is because you have undergone a major surgery which requires that you be constantly monitored and evaluated. Your bedside nurse will watch for subtle changes that indicate you may be experiencing a known complication from the surgery. Your bedside nurse will be keeping your surgeons and other members of the team informed about your progress.

Why do I need so many tubes, catheters and wires?

After surgery you will have a variety of tubes, catheters and wires in place to aid in your healing. It is important that you avoid touching these areas. The tubes will be removed as soon as it is safe to do so, but be sure to let your nurse know if any of the tubes are causing you pain or discomfort. The explanation of each tube or wire is explained below:

- **Breathing Tube**: You may wake up with a breathing tube in your mouth, and you will not be able to talk. Do not panic! This tube is important for breathing. Often it is removed within hours. In some cases, it may have to stay in for a number of days.

  While the tube is in your throat, your nurse will ask you yes-and-no questions you can answer by shaking your head. Your nurse may also provide paper and a pen so that you communicate until the breathing tube is removed. Mucus is removed from the tube by occasional suctioning. Suctioning involves sliding a smaller tube, or catheter, into the inside of the breathing tube to remove any mucus.

- Intravenous (IV) Catheters: You may wake up to find IV catheters placed in your neck, chest, arms and/or hands. These tubes provide you with fluid, medication and possibly nutrition.

- Pacer Wires: You may have 2 to 4 small wires coming from your chest wall. These wires are attached to the surface of your heart and may be used temporarily to assist your heart to beat more quickly until it recovers from the surgery.

- **Bladder Tube**: There likely will be a tube in your bladder to drain urine. This was likely inserted in the operating room. This tube is also called a urinary catheter.

- Chest Tubes: These tubes are placed during surgery to help drain blood and fluids from around the surgical sites.

How will my care be different on the step-down unit from the ICU?

The frequency of monitoring will be less, which means that you will not have one nurse who remains at your bedside throughout the day and night. Your tubes and drains will be removed throughout your recovery in the ICU and the step-down unit. However, one IV will stay in place until it's time for you to leave the hospital. This is important so that your nurses have a quick way to give you medications if there is an emergency. If you have pain or discomfort around the IV site, let your nurse know and a new IV can be placed.

Your bedside nurse on the step-down unit will continue to monitor your blood pressure, heart rate and temperature vital signs. Your nurse will also be concerned about providing opportunities for you to sleep. Nurses may "bundle care" – or coordinate as many activities as possible into a consolidated amount of time, resulting in less interruptions and more restful periods. Assisting you with bathing, toileting, ambulating, eating and taking your medications over an hour or two should allow you to get the rest you need so that you can recover more quickly.

The information from your cardiac monitoring equipment (known as telemetry) will be checked continuously throughout your hospital stay. This allows your caregivers to watch your heartbeat for irregularities or to monitor if your rate is too fast or too slow. The telemetry patches will be changed or moved every couple of days. If you feel itching around the patch, let your nurse know – another type of patch can be used that is gentler for sensitive skin.

What tests can I expect to have as I am recovering from cardiac surgery?

Several tests, procedures or images will be necessary throughout your stay. Your nurse will advise you of upcoming tests and explain why you are having the procedure.

- A chest X-ray will be obtained to determine whether the chest tube is ready to be removed. A chest X-ray is done either in your room or in the radiology department and allows your caregivers to monitor for fluid in your chest.
- An echocardiogram is done to see the way blood is flowing through your heart after surgery.
- Your blood glucose likely will be checked frequently (even if you do not have diabetes), which may require blood to be taken from your finger several times a day. Stress from surgery, or the side effects of surgery-related medications, may cause your blood glucose to rise. Research has shown that high blood glucose levels after surgery can increase your risk of infection. Insulin may be ordered to keep your blood glucose within an acceptable range.
- Your blood levels will be taken frequently while you are in the hospital. The procedure often is done early in the morning and may interrupt your sleep, but having those lab results early in the day can help your provider respond effectively to any concerns.

How will my pain be managed?

The secret to success in your recovery is walking, deep breathing and coughing, and good nutrition. If your pain is not well controlled, you may not be able to walk well, breath effectively or feel up to eating.

Your nurse will assess your pain level frequently during your stay. If your pain is not well controlled, please let your nurse know right away. Ask your nurse to provide a list of your pain medications and how often they are available.

How will getting out of bed and moving around help me after cardiac surgery?

Every patient in a hospital is at risk for a venous thromboembolism (VTE), also known as a blood clot, but this is especially true for those who have had cardiac surgery. You will be asked to wear graduated compression hose (tight white socks on your calves) or intermittent pneumatic compression sleeves (sleeves around your calf that fill with air and massage your legs). While this may be inconvenient or uncomfortable, it is important to wear one or the other as often as possible (except while bathing) to reduce your risk of VTE. If the device is uncomfortable or painful, let your nurse know and it can be reapplied or changed.

Moving and walking are important to your recovery, and your nurse will encourage you to walk at least 3 times a day. Even if you feel strong or able, the effects of some of your medications (such as blood pressure medications and diuretics/water pills) may cause you to feel dizzy when sitting up or standing. It is important to have help as you move from the bed to the chair, go to the bathroom or get up to walk, as you may have unexpected dizziness or weakness. Please talk with your nurse about when you can get up without help.

Your recovery should reflect the activities you will be doing for yourself once you are home. Your family is welcome to stay with you and participate in your care by helping you get washed up, walk and get to the chair/bed. They may also ask questions about your condition and care. Your nurse can advise the best ways your family can take an active part in your care.

What possible complications should I be aware of after cardiac surgery?

Heart surgery can lead to temporary heart rhythm changes due to trauma or irritation of the heart tissue. Some patients will need to use a temporary external pacemaker. An external pacemaker is attached to wires that have been placed in your heart through your chest during surgery. The pacemaker sends a small amount of electricity through the wires to make the heart beat. These wires may remain in place for several days.

Often, the wires are removed by the doctor or nurse practitioner at least one day prior to discharge. However, there are times that the wires are cut instead. Your nurse will provide you with special instructions if your wires have been cut. During and after the time of pacemaker wire removal, your nurse will closely monitor your vital signs to be sure you are not having a rare but serious complication called cardiac tamponade. Cardiac tamponade is bleeding around your heart. Your nurse is looking for changes in your heart rate or blood pressure in the hours after pacemaker wire removal. You will be asked to stay in bed for a period after the removal.

You may notice that you feel swollen or sweaty after your surgery. It is normal to retain fluid, and this can continue after you are discharged. You may be given medication to help rid your body of the extra fluid. If you notice that the swelling is not improving, or it is uncomfortable, let your nurse know and she/he can speak to your doctor about adjusting your medications.

Mood swings also are normal after surgery. If you find that changes in your mood or your emotions are overwhelming or difficult to manage, let your nurse know. He or she can provide resources to help you.

How should I care for my incision?

Your nurse will show you how to care for your incision while you are in the hospital. Some tips on caring for your incision after cardiac surgery include:

- Keep incisions clean, dry and open to air. Do not cover them with bandages or dressings unless it is recommended to do so because there is drainage or fluid coming from the incision.
- Refrain from using lotions or ointments on or around your incision.
- Shower with plain soap and water.
- If your stitches are not removed before discharge, they can be removed at your scheduled follow-up appointment.
- Monitor yourself for signs of infection such as fever, an increase in pain, redness, drainage or warmth on or around the incisions. If you notice this while you are in the hospital, let your nurse know right away. If you already are home, please call your doctor.

My surgery and recovery have been stressful for my family. What tips do you have to help them cope?

Families and friends play an important role in the healing process. A strong connection to family and friends helps reduce the stress of a hospitalization on the patient. The love and support family and friends provide can be as potent as medication to the healing process.

It is important for family members and friends to be aware of the toll that the patient's hospitalization may have on them. Anxiety and stress related to disruption of a normal routine are commonly experienced when a loved one is hospitalized.

There are a number of ways family members or friends can reduce their stress and anxiety related to hospital visits of a convalescing loved one. These include:

- Caring for themselves, deliberately and conscientiously - this includes eating right and continuing to exercise.
- Getting as much rest as possible. They will be spending more time visiting now that you are alert. Since you will be much more active when you are transferred to step-down, they will probably be assisting you with meals and helping you walk in the hallways as much as possible. Your loved one will also be learning how to help you recuperate once you are at home.

Here are a few things your family and friends can do to relieve stress and maintain a positive attitude when visiting the hospital:

- Walk in the halls.
- Pray in the chapel.
- Browse in stores and gift shops.
- Take advantage of any on-site music or entertainment. Many hospitals recognize the value of bringing in musicians and other performers to provide a welcome distraction.

Are there any other strategies for wellness available while I'm recovering from cardiac surgery?

The concept and practice of "complementary medicine" has been embraced by many healthcare institutions. As the title suggests, complementary therapy is used along with the therapies many consider to be traditional medicine. Complementary medicine may help you cope with, and feel better about, your treatment. It also may help reduce pain, make you feel stronger and calmer and enhance your overall quality of life.

Some types of complementary medicine are:

- Aromatherapy, which uses essential oils and other scents for the purpose of calming and relaxing the hospitalized patient.

- Pet therapy, in which animals, usually dogs, spend time with hospitalized patients
- Massage therapy, which is the manipulation of muscle using various techniques to help in the healing process and promote relaxation and well-being.
- Visualization and guided imagery, which involves focusing attention on positive objects, places or experiences that assist the patient in removing attention from pain or discomfort.
- Yoga involves stretches and low-impact physical exercise. Yoga may be used with meditation, imagery and music.
- Reiki uses a technique known as palm healing or hands-on-healing. Practitioners believe they are transferring universal energy through the palms, which they believe helps with healing.
- Meditation is a practice by which the patient trains the mind to relax through deep contemplation.
- Prayer is an act of worship or a spiritual thought, which can have positive physical and mental benefits.
- Art and music therapy use the stimulation and creative energy of the arts to improve a patient's mood, attitude and overall outlook.

What do I need to know about managing my condition safely once I go home?

On the day of your discharge, your nurse will review discharge instructions with you.

- Copies of your operative report, echocardiogram, lab results and other procedure reports often will be included for you. Share this information with your primary care doctor during your follow-up appointment, but be sure to keep a copy for your records.
- If you have any questions about medications, restrictions or your follow-up schedule, ask your nurse. Understanding what to expect once you are home is important.

- Your family should bring clothes you can comfortably travel in (including jacket and shoes) for your discharge.

Before going home, you should be able to answer "YES" to all of the following statements:

✓ I know the names, dosages and directions for taking ALL my medications that have been prescribed.

✓ I have prescriptions for all of my pills.

✓ I know how to care for my incision.

✓ I know what foods and the amounts of foods I should eat to promote good health.

✓ I know the signs and symptoms of an infection near the area where I had surgery.

✓ I know when to follow up with my doctor.

✓ I know the restrictions on my activity (walking, climbing stairs, exercise, etc.).

✓ I know when I may resume driving.

✓ I know when I may resume intimacy with my partner.

✓ I know who to call if my condition worsens or if I have a concern.

✓ I have received a referral to a social worker or case manager if I have financial or social concerns that will prevent me from obtaining medications or other home supplies.

Are there INTERNET resources where I can learn more about cardiac surgery?

National Heart, Lung and Blood Institute (What is Heart Surgery?)
http://www.nhlbi.nih.gov/health/health-topics/topics/hs/

Gastrointestinal Surgery – Intestinal Diversions

Ron Rock

You may be reading this because you or a loved one has been suffering with inflammatory bowel disease, diverticulitis or colon cancer. The disease may have progressed, resulting in increased pain or a blockage in your intestine. In order to remove the blockage or reduce your pain, you doctor has determined that you need surgery to remove all or part of your intestine.

This chapter will describe the two types of surgery which result in an ostomy. This surgery is known as an intestinal diversion which creates either a colostomy or ileostomy – a surgically created opening in your abdomen that allows waste (feces) to leave your body. This chapter will also describe your recovery in the hospital and recommendations to successfully manage your stoma.

What is a stoma?
A stoma is the end of the small or large intestine that is brought out through your abdomen during surgery. It is the new site where your waste

will leave your body. The opening itself is called a stoma. Your stoma may be temporary or permanent, and your surgeon will discuss what is needed to manage your disease.

Where will the stoma be located on my abdomen?

In order to be sure that the stoma is in the right place for all of your activities, a nurse with advanced knowledge, expertise and skill in caring for patients with ostomies will evaluate your abdomen while you are in different positions – sitting, standing and lying down – to find the best location for the stoma. These nurses use the title Wound, Ostomy, Continence Care Nurse, or WOC nurse, and are certified in this specialty. Your WOC nurse will mark the spot where the stoma will be placed with a small tattoo before surgery. A colostomy stoma is usually placed in the lower left part of the abdomen; an ileostomy stoma is usually placed in the lower right abdomen.

What is the difference between a colostomy and ileostomy?

A colostomy is where a portion of your colon or large intestine is brought to the abdomen. An ileostomy brings a portion of your small bowel known as the ileum to the abdomen. In addition to the different parts of the intestine being used to create a stoma, there is a difference in the amount or consistency of the waste coming out of the stoma. (Another term that is used for intestinal waste is stool. Stool will be the term used in the remainder of this chapter.)

The stool that drains from a colostomy is more formed, while stool from an ileostomy is more liquid.

If I have a colostomy, what is important for me to know about managing it?

Constipation can be a problem and you want to take steps to prevent it. It may be caused by lack of fiber in your diet, not drinking adequate fluids or not getting enough physical activity. There are also certain medications in which constipation is a side effect. Drink a minimum of 8 cups of fluid a day, with water being the preferable fluid of choice. You may also find it helpful to use over-the-counter laxatives. Discuss this with your surgeon prior to taking a laxative.

You may need to manage your colostomy with routine irrigations of tap water to improve and regulate bowel function. If so, your WOC nurse will teach you the correct technique and ask that you practice this skill while you are in the hospital so that you gain confidence.

If I have an ileostomy, what is important for me to know about managing it?

Protect your skin around your stoma. Ileostomies can produce up to a liter of output a day. The output contains a large amount of digestive enzymes, which can be extremely irritating to your skin.

Drink at least 8 to 10 glasses of water daily to prevent dehydration. Limit your intake of caffeine and alcohol as these beverages can dehydrate you. Because you have an ileostomy, the fluids that would have normally been absorbed by the large intestines are eliminated in your pouch. As a result, it is important for you to take precautions against dehydration. You will be instructed to increase your daily fluid intake by 1 to 2 glasses of water per day.

Eat high fiber foods. Fiber adds bulk to the stool. High fiber foods include bran cereals, fresh fruits, vegetables (raw and cooked), whole wheat breads and whole grains.

Be alert for signs of blockage. These symptoms include no output from the ileostomy, high-volume liquid output with a foul smell, cramping pain, abdominal swelling and possibly nausea and vomiting.

Talk with your doctor and pharmacist about the medications you were taking before your surgery. Since you have an ileostomy, some of the medications previously prescribed will not be absorbed properly. This is especially true for coated tablets or extended release tablets. Whenever possible, you should use liquid forms of medications for better absorption.

What can I expect when I wake up from surgery?

As you wake up from surgery, you may feel some discomfort over the abdominal area. Your bedside nurse will monitor your vital signs and pain level. It is important to let your nurse know how you are tolerating your pain and to request pain medication BEFORE you become too uncomfortable. You may have a pain pump which you will control by pushing a button to dispense medication into your Intravenous line (IV) when you need it. The pain pump has a maximum rate and will not give you more than is safe.

You will receive fluids through your IV line for several days. Your IV will remain until you are eating sufficiently and drinking without any complaints of nausea and vomiting.

You may have a tube in your nose that goes in your stomach and is attached to a suction machine. The tube may cause some irritation at the back of throat. The purpose of the tube is to prevent you from feeling nauseated as your bowels recover from the surgery. You will not be able to drink fluids while the tube is in your nose. You may be permitted ice chips.

You may also have a tube that is inserted into your bladder that will drain urine. This tube, called a urinary catheter, will be taken out as soon as possible after surgery.

Your stoma will have a pouch to collect stool. You will learn how to manage your stoma as you recover in the hospital.

What is an ostomy pouch?

An ostomy pouch is a medical device applied over your stoma to collect your stool. It is made of heavy duty plastic and resembles a bag. The pouch is selected and fitted to your body by your WOC nurse.

The pouch is usually changed every 3 to 4 days. Your skin will be protected from stool with the correct pouching system. Pouches are emptied in the commode when they are between one-third and one-half full. The pouch is odor-proof and waterproof and lays flat against your body. This allows the pouch to be disguised under clothing, so that nobody will be able to tell you are wearing a pouch.

Your WOC nurse will teach you how to change your pouch after your surgery. You will have 1 to 2 lessens, depending on the length of your stay. A home care nurse can also give you ostomy lessons at home. These lessons are recommended to help you improve your skills and feel more confident in taking care of yourself.

Before you leave the hospital, you will be given a several-week supply of pouches to take home and a prescription so that you can order your own pouches. Patients are responsible for ordering supplies after discharge. The home care ostomy nurses can help you with the ordering process. Most or all of the cost of the pouches is covered by insurance. You can check your coverage by calling your insurance company. Ostomy supplies are usually billed under the category of "Durable Medical Equipment."

How often do I need to change my pouch?

Your pouch needs to be changed on a regular basis – every 4 to 7days. It will need to be changed more frequently if you have:

- Leaking
- Itching or burning under your pouch

How do I manage odor and gas?

After surgery odor and gas are common concerns with an ostomy. The pouches are odor proof. You will be taught how to keep the end of the pouch clean so that it does not become a source of odor. When you empty the pouch, odor is normal; room sprays or pouch deodorants can be used to minimize odor.

Gas control may require you to modify your diet, and over-the-counter gas reducing products are important to reduce the amount of gas that is produced. Common foods that may cause odor or gas in some individuals include beans, cabbage, cauliflower, brussels sprouts, broccoli, garlic, onions and asparagus.

What changes do I need to make to my diet?

After your surgery, you will have some swelling in your abdomen. This is normal. You will be prescribed a special diet known as a soft GI diet. While you are on this diet, you will not be able to eat raw fruits and vegetables for approximately 4 to 6 weeks.

Right after surgery, the stool that you produce will be mostly liquid. Certain foods, such as pasta, mashed potatoes and applesauce, will help thicken the stool. After six weeks, you will be able to start adding different foods back into your diet one at a time and in moderation. It is important to chew your food thoroughly. It is also important to eat at regular times and not skip meals. Skipping meals can cause more gas.

Some foods are not digested by the body. These include corn, mushrooms and peanuts, and you may notice them in your pouch if you eat them. This is completely normal.

Eating should be enjoyable. Eat a wide range of different foods. If you have other medical conditions, such as heart disease or diabetes, you may need additional nutrition guidance. Ask to see a dietitian so that your diet questions and nutritional concerns can be addressed.

What am I able to do after surgery?

Increase your activities a little each day. There are generally no restrictions to walking, climbing stairs or riding in a car.

Do not lift anything heavier than a gallon of milk for the first 6 weeks after surgery to prevent a hernia. After 6 weeks, you can resume most activities safely with minimal or no changes. For example, you may bathe or shower with the pouch on or off. Changes in your clothes are generally not needed.

Most sports activities can be resumed as well, with the exception of extreme contact sports, which could potentially damage the stoma. The addition of a belt or binder is helpful in maintaining a pouch seal during activity and perspiration. Ask your surgeon how much you may lift and when you can go back to work.

Are there traveling restrictions since I have a stoma?

There are no traveling restrictions. However, it is important for you to take extra supplies. If you are flying, place your stoma supplies in your carry-on luggage. Cut and prepare your stoma appliance before packing, because it will be difficult to prepare your pouch in the very restricted space on an airplane restroom should you need to do so. Book an aisle seat so you have easier access to the restroom. Avoid exposing the supplies to extreme temperatures, which may affect how well the pouch will stick to your skin. This could cause your pouch to leak.

Are there restrictions to resuming intimacy with my partner?

Check with your doctor before resuming sexual activity. This is a concern for most patients who have undergone ostomy surgery. As you recover from surgery and begin to resume an intimate relationship, give yourself and your partner time. Counseling to address questions regarding your sexual activity and partner response could be critical to rehabilitation of the ostomy patient. Empty the pouch, and make sure the seal of the pouch is intact before engaging in sexual activity. In addition, it may be helpful to use special lingerie or cummerbunds to conceal and secure the pouch.

What are symptoms that require a call to my doctor or my WOC nurse?

- Your stoma is swollen and is more than a half inch larger than normal.
- Your stoma is pulling in, below the skin level.
- Your stoma is bleeding more than normal.
- Your stoma has turned purple, black or white.
- Your stoma is leaking often or draining fluid.
- You have a discharge from the stoma that smells bad.
- You have any signs of being dehydrated, which means there is not enough water in your body. Some signs are dry mouth, urinating less often and feeling lightheaded or weak.
- You have less waste than usual in your pouch.
- You have a fever.
- You experience any pain.
- You have diarrhea that is not going away.

Call your WOC nurse if the skin around your stoma:

- Pulls back
- Is red or raw
- Has a rash

- Is dry
- Hurts or burns
- Swells or pushes out
- Has white, gray, brown or dark red bumps on it
- Has bumps around a hair follicle that are filled with pus
- Has sores with uneven edges

Before going home, you should be able to answer "YES" to all of the following statements:

✓ I know the names, dosages and directions for taking ALL my medications that have been prescribed.

✓ I have a prescription for any new medications.

✓ I have a prescription for my ostomy equipment.

✓ I know how to reorder my ostomy equipment.

✓ I know what foods to eat and what foods to avoid to minimize gas.

✓ I know how much fluid to drink to prevent dehydration.

✓ I know what I can do to protect the skin around my stoma when I change my pouch.

✓ I know the signs of an intestinal blockage and actions to take if that occurs.

✓ I know the changes in my stoma that require a call to my doctor.

✓ I know the restrictions on my activity (walking, climbing stairs, exercise, etc.).

✓ I know when I can resume driving.

✓ I know when I can resume intimacy with my partner.

Are there INTERNET resources
where I can learn more about living with an ostomy?

Cancercare
www.cancer.org

Colon Cancer Alliance (CCA)
www.ccalliance.org

Crohn's & Colitis Foundation of America (CCFA)
www.ccfa.org

Friends of Ostomates Worldwide (FOW-USA)
www.fowusa.org

International Ostomy Association (IOA)
www.ostomyinternational.org

United Ostomy Associations of America (UOAA)
www.ostomy.org

Wound, Ostomy, Continence Nurses Society
www.wocn.org

Young Ostomates United
www.youincorg.au/

Orthopedic Surgery

Lydia Booher

Living with joint pain can be very debilitating. Having lived with this pain for years, you have developed strategies for managing your pain, swelling and stiffness in your joints. You may have tried numerous conservative treatments before deciding that joint replacement surgery is necessary to help decrease your pain, increase your mobility and improve your quality of life.

Your orthopedic surgeon will have described the surgical procedure, pain management techniques, postoperative course and your rehabilitation phase before you are admitted to the hospital. This chapter will discuss the nursing care you will receive in the hospital and the patient education you will need to aid in your recovery.

How will my pain be managed?

Managing your pain is a priority for your entire caregiver team. Your bedside nurse will ask you to rate your pain on a scale from 0 to 10, with 0 being no pain and 10 being the worst pain you have experienced. Your nurses will reassess your pain after administering your pain medication and will communicate your pain regimen and relief with the entire caregiver team.

It is important to know that it may not always be possible to achieve a 0 out of 10 pain rating, but great care and attention will be spent on your pain management. Listening to music can also be an effective pain reduction pain strategy. Pain will be managed through multiple methods and routes (i.e. by mouth, through intravenous line (IV) and/or nerve block).

Pain management for three specific surgeries is described below:

- **Total Hip Replacement:** Immediately after your total hip replacement, your pain will be managed by medication given through your intravenous (IV) line. Once you are able to eat you will begin to take pain medication in pill or liquid form. Often, oral and IV medicines are alternated based on your pain score.
- **Total Shoulder Replacement:** A nerve catheter is inserted close to the surgery site to block pain. You will also receive intravenous and oral pain medications. You will be taught how to care for the nerve catheter by your bedside nurse. The catheter will remain in place when you are discharged unless there is a contraindication for its use at home.
- **Total Knee Replacement:** A nerve block will be used to complement intravenous and oral pain medications. The nerve block may be a single shot or a continuous infusion. It provides pain relief for 48 to 72 hours. Usually, the nerve catheter is discontinued on the first or second postoperative day. The nerve block only numbs the top of the knee. If you have severe pain to back of the knee, you need to notify your bedside nurse.

What if I am still in pain after my nurse gives me medication?

An important principle in effective pain management is to "stay on top of your pain." Your caregivers want you to ask for pain medication before your pain becomes "unbearable." This way your pain can be effectively managed.

In addition, your nurse will check in with you after you have received your pain medication to make sure that you are comfortable.

Patients with chronic pain may experience more severe pain postoperatively. If you suffer from chronic pain, share this with your surgeon at your preoperative visit so that a pain plan can be established.

I am worried about dislocating my new joint after my surgery. What can I do to prevent that from happening?

Your bedside nurse and physical therapist will instruct you on proper alignment and safety precautions following surgery. If you have undergone a hip replacement it is important to keep the (abduction) pillow in between your legs at least for the first 24 hours. This keeps the leg from rolling inward and dislocating the new hip. Avoid crossing your legs or bending your knee more than 90 degrees. To avoid dislocating the new hip, do not bend down to pick anything up from the floor. You will be given a tool that will help you.

If you have undergone a shoulder replacement, the operated side will be placed in a sling. It will be removed when you work with the occupational therapist. Your shoulder and arm should be well supported while you are lying in bed. Your bedside nurse will make sure that you are using the sling correctly.

When will I get out of bed for the first time?

Activity after total joint replacement is an important stepping stone toward recovery. Your muscles need to be strengthened as early as possible after surgery as they may be weak due to restricted mobility caused by pain before surgery. Early mobility also assists with the prevention of blood clots, constipation and difficulty urinating.

After surgery, you will be assisted by your bedside nurse and physical therapist to sit on the side of the bed with your feet dangling. You may even be assisted to walk in the hallway. Your bedside nurse and nursing assistant will remind you frequently to call for help if you want to get out of bed. You might be weak or drowsy due to anesthesia or pain medications. It is essential that you notify your nurse that you want to get up, especially if he/she is not there to assist you. Do not overestimate your feeling of strength or ability. You have just undergone a surgical procedure, and this is a time when many patients fall by accident.

Will I have to use a bedpan, or can I get up to go to the bathroom?

Possibly. Although you may feel that it is safe to get out of bed by yourself or with the assistance of a loved one, this is **STRONGLY DISCOURAGED.** You may be assisted to a bedside commode on the day of surgery if you are not dizzy. If not, your caregivers will assist you onto a bedpan.

Will I be on a restricted diet?

If you are not nauseous and are able to tolerate fluids, your first meal will be a light meal. Eating healthy foods is important to your recovery and to wound healing. If you miss a meal because you were sleeping, ask your bedside nurse about arranging for a snack. If your hospital has "Room Service" or "Meals upon Request," missing a meal should not be a problem. If you need assistance with opening items on your tray, share this with your nurse. Preventing constipation is an important goal for patients undergoing joint replacement surgeries. Please include high fiber content in your meals, such as high fiber cereal, prunes and prune juice, and drink a lot of fluids.

Will I be able to sit in a chair to eat my meals?

You may not be able to eat your first meal after surgery in a chair because of the effects of anesthesia. It will depend on what time you are admitted to your room and meal time. It is highly encouraged to get out of bed and eat meals in a chair from the first postoperative day until discharge. Discuss this request with your bedside nurse.

Why do I have to wear special stockings?

People who undergo total knee and hip replacements are at very high risk for developing blood clots. It is very important to wear the intermittent pneumatic compression (IPC) stockings for a significant part of the days. The stockings keep the blood moving and decrease the chance of developing blood clots. The IPC stockings will be removed while you are walking and bathing. You need to wear them even while sitting in the chair. Many patients complain of the noise from the pump or sweating caused by the stockings. You can take a brief break from wearing the stockings but it is important to put them back on. Remember that the IPC stockings cannot help unless they are on your legs.

Will I have to take a blood thinner?

After a total hip or knee replacement you are at risk for developing a blood clot. The danger of a blood clot is that it could travel to your lungs or your brain. You may need to take a blood thinner medication, also referred to as an anticoagulant, to prevent a blood clot. You may need to take this medication at home after discharge. Blood thinning medications may be given as an injection or in pill form. Your bedside nurse will teach you how to take these medications safely and explain any potential side effects.

What is the rehabilitation after joint surgery?

Your surgeon will have discussed the need for rehabilitation/physical therapy when you consented to the surgery. Your physical therapist is integral to your recovery and will instruct you on the specific exercises necessary to optimize your joint replacement. A physical therapist will meet with you in your hospital room to assess you and discuss your exercise regimen.

Remember that your physical therapy and strengthening exercises will help you gain greater mobility and ensure an easier recovery following surgery. It is highly recommended that you continue therapy treatment for the recommended timeframe prescribed by your physical therapist.

Do I need to go to a rehabilitation facility after my surgery?

Your surgeon may determine that a rehabilitation facility will be the best choice for your recovery after discharge from the hospital. At the rehabilitation center, you will have designated time with a physical therapist and occupational therapist to help you regain your strength and learn about your exercises and the precautions that you'll need to follow. Your length of stay at this facility is approximately 5 to 14 days.

What do I need to know before I go home?

Before going home, you should be able to answer "YES" to all of the following statements:

✓ I know the names, dosages and directions for taking ALL medications that have been prescribed.

✓ I know the exercises I need to perform daily to increase my strength, balance and endurance.

✓ I know what my physical therapy schedule will be and where I will be receiving therapy.

✓ I know the restrictions on my activity – walking, climbing stairs, getting in and out of a car, etc.

✓ I know what modifications I need to make to my home to prevent falls.

✓ I know how to get up from a seated position safely (Total Hip Replacement).

✓ I know how to safely perform Range of Motion (ROM) exercises (Total Knee Replacement).

✓ I know what foods and the amounts of foods I should eat to assist with healing.

✓ I know how to inject my blood thinner if I am going home on an injectable medication.

✓ I know what foods to avoid if I am taking a blood thinner.

✓ I know when I can resume driving.

✓ I know when I can resume intimacy with my partner.

✓ I know when and whom to call about symptoms of increased pain, wound infection, swelling or bleeding.

Are there INTERNET resources where I can learn more about arthritis and joint replacement?

Academy of Nutrition and Dietetics

www.eatright.org

American Academy of Orthopedic Surgeons

www.aaos.org

American Association of Hip and Knee Surgeons

www.aahks.org

American Council on Exercise

www.acefitness.org

American Physical Therapy

www.apta.org

Arthritis Foundation

www.arthritis.org

Centers for Disease Control and Prevention
www.cdc.gov

Part Five:

Partnering with Your Caregivers in the Care of Special Populations

"Within the child lies the fate of the future."
Maria Montessori, MD

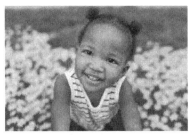
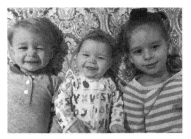
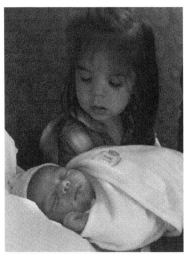
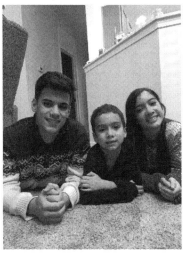

Pregnancy

Ann Roach

Congratulations, you are about to have a baby! Lots of wonderful events take place in a hospital, but having a baby and taking your baby home with you is one of the most joyful events. Employees, other patients and their visitors are also overjoyed when they see you with your baby. When a baby is born, most hospitals will play a little piece of music – usually part of Brahms' lullaby – throughout the entire hospital. Even the sickest patients smile when they hear that music being played. Everybody likes to celebrate babies!

You have probably attended childbirth classes and read a lot about pregnancy. This chapter is meant to supplement those resources and will provide good reminders about what you can expect while in the hospital.

How do I mentally prepare to give birth?
There are only 2 ways for your baby to arrive. The first way is through the vagina, also known as the birth canal, and the second way is through a surgical incision in your abdomen. This is a cesarean section or more commonly known as a C section. The recovery for each is a bit different for the mom, although recovery is definitely a bit faster when the baby arrives

through the vagina. However, the end result is what matters. Everybody wants a healthy mom and a healthy baby.

Labor is a process. Labor is work. Labor is uncomfortable. Very few moms have ever said "I loved being in labor. It was so much fun!" In fact, they are more likely to say "I was in labor for days and had to push for hours and hours". Have you ever noticed that the labor stories of your friends and family members tend to grow a little bit bigger each time they repeat them?

Think of giving birth as taking an entire day – 24 hours. It is a birthday after all, and birthdays are absolutely very special days. Think of your baby's day of birth as one very LONG day. It never happens like it does on TV or in the movies. It WILL take longer than half an hour, but it usually takes less than 24 hours. Your nurses, doctors and midwives are there to help you bring your baby into the world. They all want you to relax as much as possible, to trust your body and to help you and your baby journey safely through labor and your hospital stay.

Do I need a support person to help me with labor?

Your support in labor plays an important role in your comfort. Most of the time the major support person is also the person who will be helping to raise the baby. They are fathers, partners or other family members. They can help you by:

- Rubbing your back
- Giving you ice chips
- Providing distraction
- Helping you with your breathing
- Encouraging you

What does the nurse do to help me give birth?

When you are in labor, your nurse is your advocate. Your nurse will:

- Suggest lots of different ways to cope with the discomforts of labor and celebrate with you when the baby is born.
- Help you breathe and relax. A big part of labor is being patient and "letting it happen." If you are relaxed, your breathing is easier. If your breathing is easier, oxygen is moving to your muscles, and muscles with oxygen are comfortable; you will experience much less labor discomfort!
- Encourage you to get out of bed and rock in a rocker, sit on an exercise ball, dance with your partner, get into the shower to relax or use the Jacuzzi tub for labor comfort.
- Assess your energy level. A lot of laboring moms feel that they must entertain visitors, and it can be exhausting. Your nurse will be happy to run interference for you and have family members wait in the waiting room for a little bit longer so that you can take a break from entertaining and focus on yourself.
- Recognize when it is getting a little bit tough for you and move on to support you with "medical" options that are available to you.
- Collaborate with your doula if you have chosen to include one in your birth plan. (Doulas are specially-trained individuals who are hired by moms to provide labor support before arriving to the hospital in labor. Doulas help the mom design the birth plan.)
- Monitor your contractions and blood pressure.
- Coach you through the "pushing phase."
- Celebrate with you once your baby is born.

What is a doula?

A doula, also called a "birth attendant," provides physical and emotional support to the mother and her partner before, during and after childbirth.

How will my pain be managed?

You can help the nurses by letting them know what makes you comfortable. Do you love music, or do you need absolute quiet to relax? Your nurse is an expert in creating the environment that will help you labor best.

Pain medication is another option for staying comfortable during labor. The medication is delivered by an epidural (a catheter that is placed in your back) by an anesthesiologist or a certified registered nurse anesthetist (CRNA). This medication decreases the sensation in the lower part of your body.

What is a fetal monitor?

An important part of labor for the nurse is also keeping an eye on how your baby is doing. Since your belly doesn't come with a window that lets nurses watch the baby directly, they keep track of how the baby is doing by listening to his or her heartbeat. This is easy to do with a fetal monitor.

The monitor on your belly acts just like a stethoscope, and the entire room can hear the baby's heartbeat. The downside is that when you are being continuously monitored you are linked to the machine by a cord. This makes it a bit hard to dance or walk around the room and makes it impossible to relax in the tub.

Sometimes, the baby can be monitored with a hand- held monitor, which will let you move around a lot more. Movement in labor helps the baby move down and out of the birth canal a lot easier.

How does the nurse or doctor know when I am having a contraction?

Besides you telling us, your nurse and doctor will know you are having contractions because of a second monitor that will be placed on your belly. This second monitor traces your contractions and provides a record of your contractions throughout your labor. Uterine contractions are the strong muscle movements that bring your baby to you. They are also what make labor pretty uncomfortable. Your nurse will review your contractions for intensity and timing – how long each one lasts and the time between contractions.

Will I be able to eat when I am in labor?

When you are in labor, your nurse will assess your thirst level and provide clear liquids such as water, apple juice, gelatin and ice. You are discouraged from eating while you are in active labor because food is not digested as quickly. In addition, most moms are not very hungry as they are concentrating on giving birth to their baby.

Most moms will have an intravenous (IV) line to provide fluid and give medications. Blood work can be drawn from your IV when it is first started, and it can be used to give you additional pain medications. A drug called Pitocin may be given if your labor slows down or your contractions are not moving the baby down the birth canal. Your doctor will discuss the need for this medication should the occasion arise.

What is "kangaroo care"?

If your baby has been born vaginally, the baby will be placed immediately on your chest to promote bonding between mom and baby. This is called "kangaroo care". It also helps to regulate the baby's temperature.

Watch the magic unfold as your baby relaxes, stretches and becomes very comfortable in your arms. It also puts the baby in the perfect position to receive their first feeding. Should your baby be delivered by cesarean section, nurses will make sure that your baby receives the benefit of skin-to-skin contact with you or with your partner in the operating room.

What does the term postpartum mean?

This marks the time after you have the baby. It is a time for getting to know and love your baby. It is also important to allow your body to rest. You are still going through some pretty remarkable changes to return to your pre-pregnant state (and it is going to take weeks). In the hospital, you now have some time to get to know your little one while you also recover from labor. Eat good food, drink lots of water, nap when your baby naps, and look at, listen to and hold your baby. Skin to skin bonding is still wonderful to practice throughout your hospital stay.

Nurses will be by your hospital room very often to check on the size of your uterus by pushing gently on your abdomen. They will also check your vaginal bleeding. (You should still expect some bleeding after you give birth.) They will be rounding or checking on you at least every hour during the day and about every 2 hours during the night. This is a perfect opportunity for you to ask questions or watch how the nurse swaddles and holds your baby. Babies really do not come with instructions. You might need help in learning everything from how to hold your baby to how to get a t-shirt on a baby.

If you have had a cesarean section, you have had an operation. Learn how to care for your incision while you are in the hospital so that you can care for it at home. There are also some tips and tricks on how to hold or breast-feed your baby while staying comfortable after surgery.

Nurses want you to keep your baby in your hospital room with you. The time immediately after birth is a very special time. The more time you spend with your baby, the quicker you will learn what all the small noises mean. You will recognize when your baby is getting hungry and when the baby just seems to be stretching. You will soon find that your baby knows you and recognizes your voice and scent.

Your breast milk is the perfect food for your baby. If you choose to breast-feed your baby, your nurses will help you. You may be visited by a lactation consultant who can give you specialized breastfeeding instructions or help you solve specific problems. Learning to breastfeed is a lot like learning to dance. You hear the music, and caregivers can teach you the basic steps of the dance, but the two people involved develop their own rhythm with a little patience and practice and then it looks effortless.

Why does my baby stay in the room with me instead of the nursery?

It is best practice to allow babies to stay in the room with their mothers. This helps you get to know your baby and respond to cries or signals of discomfort. Your baby needs to sleep safely in his or her own crib. Please do not allow your baby to sleep in the bed with you. The safest place for babies to sleep is on their backs in the bassinette. New mothers are often exhausted. If you feel tired, it is best to place the baby in the bassinette or allow another adult to hold the baby while you rest. Your nurse wants you to nap when the baby is napping, but not in the same bed.

The ABCs for safe sleeping for babies:

> A = Alone
> B= On their Backs
> C= In a Crib

What if the unexpected happens and my baby needs extra care?

The neonatal intensive care unit is a place in the hospital that cares for babies that need assistance immediately after birth. If your baby has trouble breathing or eating, he or she may be in this unit. Everything about a premature baby is special, from their skin to their brain, and they need specialized care so they can continue to grow and develop. You will be meeting more caregivers if your baby needs to spend time in this unit. Please refer to the chapter on the newborns admitted to the neonatal intensive care unit for more information.

What if I am hospitalized during my pregnancy?

Pregnant women still get sick. They get the flu, they may need gall bladder surgery, or they may fall. What is different is that they have a baby on board and that requires a little bit more attention. If you are hospitalized for reasons that do not involve being pregnant, your obstetrician or midwife will be involved in your care.

Most of the time that you are hospitalized during pregnancy is for reasons related to the pregnancy. It is really tough to be in the hospital. You are away from your family, your job and your friends. Your nurses will help you find ways to cope with being hospitalized while they also keep a close watch on your health and the health and growth of your unborn baby.

What do I need to know about going home with my baby?

Plan for your discharge or "going home day" before you arrive at the hospital. Your baby will need to travel home in a properly installed, age appropriate car seat. Many fire and police stations have specially-trained staff who can help ensure your car seat is properly installed before the baby is born.

You need to have a safe place for your baby to sleep when you arrive home. This may be a crib, bassinette or portable crib.

Before going home, you should be able to answer "YES" to all of the following statements:

> ✓ I know the names, dosages and directions for taking ALL my medications that have been prescribed.

✓ I know when and how to bathe my baby and care for his or her umbilical cord.

✓ I know how to care for my baby's penis if he was circumcised.

✓ I have a thermometer, and I know how to take my baby's temperature.

✓ I know that I should call my baby's pediatrician if my baby appears to be in pain, has a fever or is not wetting diapers.

✓ I know how much vaginal bleeding to expect and when to notify my doctor or midwife if my vaginal bleeding becomes excessive or painful.

✓ I have a scheduled appointment with my baby's pediatrician.

✓ I have a scheduled appointment with my obstetrician or midwife.

✓ I know the limitations for my activity to aide in my recovery.

✓ I know what foods I should avoid if I am breastfeeding.

✓ I know how to contact a lactation consultant for questions or issues during breastfeeding.

✓ I know how much water I should drink to stay hydrated.

✓ I know how to keep my baby safe – no sleeping in bed with parent, no shaking the baby, no transporting the baby without a car seat.

✓ I know to put my baby to bed on his or her back.

✓ I know who I can call for support if I feel stressed, overwhelmed or blue

✓ I know how to recognize the signs of postpartum depression, including sadness that does not go away, feelings of hopelessness and anger or resentment toward the baby

✓ I know when I can resume intimacy with my spouse or partner

Are there INTERNET resources where I can learn more about pregnancy and childbirth?

International Childbirth Education Association
http://www.icea.org/

The American College of Nurse-Midwives
http://www.midwife.org/

The American Congress of Obstetricians and Gynecologists
http://www.acog.org/Patients

United States Breastfeeding Committee
http://www.usbreastfeeding.org/

Newborns Admitted to the Neonatal Intensive Care Unit

Tina DiFiore

This chapter is written for parents of infants who are admitted to neonatal intensive care units. A neonatal intensive care unit (NICU) is an intensive care unit that provides care to sick and preterm infants. The NICU setting may be intimidating and confusing, and families often need help coping during their baby's stay in the NICU.

Why would a baby be admitted to the NICU?

The majority of babies admitted to NICU are premature. A baby is considered premature if they are born before 38 week's gestation, or more than 2 weeks early. We often refer to these babies as 'preemies.' One in every eight babies born in the U.S. is born premature. Those born very early or who are very sick may experience a hospital stay that lasts weeks or months.

The birth of a premature or sick baby can be a very difficult time for parents and families. No family is prepared for the crisis of a premature birth. It is understandable to be concerned about your baby and the uncertain future.

Is it normal to feel emotional or overwhelmed when my baby is in the NICU?

Parents often experience grief, fear and anxiety while their baby is in the hospital. Parents also report feeling less effective as a parent or out of control. Some even begin to feel more like visitors than parents to their child or children. It is important to remember that even at this early stage parents and families are very important members of the caregiving team.

Stress often prevents parents from absorbing all the information given to them. In the NICU you will be given information from many different people. Therefore, we recommend having a journal or notebook to write down questions and instructions that have been provided. Also, remember that you may need to hear an answer several times before you are able to understand it.

It is OK to ask family or friends for support at home while you are at the hospital. Grandparents and other close family or friends may take turns caring for older children or doing household chores.

What is family-centered care?

We encourage parents to participate fully in the care of their baby. We call this family-centered care. This means that parents are encouraged to spend as much time as possible in their infant's room. Every day, your infant's caregiving team will complete rounds at the bedside and discuss your infant's condition, progress and changes to the plan of care. You are encouraged to participate in the discussion and to ask questions. If you are not available, your doctor or nurse practitioner will reach you by phone to update you and answer your questions. As a parent, you are your child's advocate. Rounds are an ideal time to become familiar with the plan of care as well as ask questions.

The NICU caregiving team is there to not only to care for your baby, but to also help you cope and learn to care for your child. They offer guidance. Learning to care for your baby in the protected environment of the NICU is very important. The nurse will teach you what you need to know about caring for your baby, what you need to do while in the NICU and why doing this is important. They will show you how to hold, feed, console and diaper your baby. They will offer feedback so that you gain confidence in providing the physical care your baby requires.

Remember that even the smallest, most premature infant is unique and has the ability to feel and communicate. The first time you see your infant remember that your baby may be very small and thin. Their skin may be red. Jerky movements are common. If your baby has a breathing tube, you will not be able to hear him or her cry.

How should I keep track of my baby's progress?

Keep track of your baby's progress on paper or a journal. Preterm infants usually make subtle changes and improvements, so having a written record will help you identify the improvements and cope with a potentially long hospitalization. Many families have said that a blank calendar page is the best way to accomplish this. This will help you see not only your baby's progress, but will help you learn to care for your baby and identify your baby's unique personality.

Avoid comparing your baby to one in the next crib or room. Each baby is an individual and therefore progresses at his or her own rate. Talk to the nursing staff to help you learn how to support his or her individual strengths.

Celebrate you and your baby's progress, especially if your baby will be in the NICU for an extended period of time.

How should I interact with my baby?

- Touch gently without stroking. Learn how to cuddle your baby with your hands. This may be referred to as facilitated tucking.
- Visit your baby when he or she is awake. All babies have alert times. Try to maximize your visitation and plan your visit around this time.
- Practice not looking at the monitors.
- Read to your baby.
- Talk or sing to your baby. All babies recognize their parents' voices.
- Watch carefully for your baby's cues. Your baby will show you when he or she is comfortable or upset.
- Sleep with a soft diaper, and then bring it in for your baby to smell when you are not here. The most developed sense for newborns is their sense of smell.

What are the most important concerns in the development of premature infants?

There are several concerns related to premature infants, including nutrition and growth, infection and respiratory problems.

Nutrition and Growth

Premature babies have special nutritional needs because they grow at a faster rate than full-term babies do. Additionally, their digestive systems are immature. These two factors provide special challenges and opportunities in providing nutrition to preterm infants.

Mother's milk is the best food for babies. The American Academy of Pediatrics recommends feeding your baby only breast milk for the first six months of his or her life. Breast milk contains anti-bodies to protect your baby against infections, help protect your baby's stomach and intestines from harmful bacteria, promote the development of the brain and nervous system, and decrease the chances of your baby having allergies, asthma or ear infections.

If your baby is big enough to coordinate their sucking, swallowing and breathing, the best way to initiate breast feeding is to put the baby directly to the breast. Breast feeding can be challenging for new mothers. The NICU nurses or a lactation consultant will help you. Lactation consultants are nurses who have additional training and certification in helping mothers breast feed.

If your baby is unable to go to the breast, we recommend that you obtain a hospital grade breast pump. The pump will mimic your baby sucking and help you obtain your milk so that it can be stored or fed to your baby. Research has demonstrated that it is important to begin pumping within the first 6 hours after you deliver your baby in order to establish an adequate supply of breast milk.

If feeding by mouth is not possible, breast milk can be pumped by the mother and fed to the premature baby through a tube that goes from the baby's nose or mouth into the stomach. Other options for feeding include pasteurized human breast milk from a milk bank, which is considered a safe alternative. Formula also may be given to babies whose mothers are not able to provide breast milk when donor breast milk is not available.

Breast milk has an advantage over formula because it contains antibodies that help fight infection and promote growth. Special fortifiers may be added to breast milk (or to formula, if breastfeeding is not desired) because premature infants have higher vitamin and mineral needs than full-term infants.

Nearly all premature babies receive additional calcium and phosphorus either by adding fortifier to breast milk or directly through special formulas. The baby's blood chemicals and minerals – such as blood glucose (sugar), salt, potassium, calcium, phosphate and magnesium – are monitored regularly, and the baby's diet is adjusted to keep these substances within a normal range.

Some preemies who are very small or very sick cannot use their digestive system to process food. These babies require intravenous (IV) nutrition – called TPN, or total parenteral nutrition – made up of fats, proteins, sugars and nutrients. TPN is given through a small tube inserted into a large vein through the baby's skin.

Infection

Infection is a big threat to premature babies because they're less able than full-term infants to fight germs that can cause serious illness. Infections can develop before birth, during the birth process or after birth. Practically any body part can become infected. Reducing the risk of infection is why frequent hand washing is necessary in the NICU.

Bacterial infections can be treated with antibiotics. Other medications are prescribed to treat viral and fungal infections.

Respiratory problems

One of the most common and immediate problems facing an infant born premature is difficulty breathing. Many things can cause breathing difficulties in premature infants, but the most common is respiratory distress syndrome (RDS).

In RDS, the baby's immature lungs do not produce enough of an important substance called surfactant. Surfactant allows the inner surface of the lungs to expand properly when the infant goes from the womb to breathing air after birth. Fortunately, RDS is treatable and many infants do quite well.

When premature delivery cannot be stopped, most pregnant women can be given medication just before delivery to hasten the production of surfactant in the infant's lungs and help prevent RDS. Then, immediately after birth and several times later, surfactant can be given to the baby if needed.

Although most premature babies who lack surfactant will require a breathing machine, or ventilator, for a while, the use of surfactant has greatly decreased the amount of time they spend on the ventilator.

What can I expect after my baby leaves the NICU?

Premature babies often require special care after leaving the NICU, sometimes in a high-risk newborn clinic or early intervention program. In addition to the regular well-child visits that all infants receive, premature infants receive periodic developmental, hearing and eye examinations.

Careful attention is paid to the development of the nervous system. This includes the achievement of motor skills like smiling, sitting and walking, as well as the positioning and strength of the muscles.

Speech and behavioral development also are important areas during follow-up. Some premature infants may need speech therapy or physical therapy as they grow up.

Family support is also important. Caring for a premature infant is even more demanding than caring for a full-term baby, so high-risk clinics pay special attention to the needs of the family as a whole.

Before taking your baby home, you should be able to answer "YES" to all of the following statements:

✓ I know when to call 911.

✓ I know the names, dosages and directions for giving ALL medications that have been prescribed for my child.

✓ I have prescriptions for all the medications that have been prescribed for my baby.

✓ I have a thermometer, and I know how to take my baby's temperature.

✓ I know that I should call my baby's pediatrician if my baby appears to be in pain, has a fever or is not wetting diapers.

✓ I know how to use the monitoring equipment that may be sent home with my baby.

✓ I know how to put my baby to bed in a crib to be safe.

✓ I know how to place my baby in her car seat.

✓ I know how to position my baby to minimize breathing difficulties.

✓ I know how to protect my baby from an infection.

✓ I know when my baby's follow-up appointments are scheduled, or I know how to schedule my child's follow-up appointments.

✓ I have received a referral to a social worker or case manager if I have financial or social concerns that will prevent me from obtaining medications or services needed for my child's follow-up care

Are there INTERNET resources where I can learn more about premature babies and the NICU?

American Academy of Pediatrics
www.healthychildren.org

Centers for Disease Control and Prevention, Life Stages and Populations http://www.cdc.gov/features/lifestages.html

March of Dimes
www.marchofdimes.org

Pebbles of Hope
www.pebblesofhope.org

The Surgical Newborn in the Neonatal Intensive Care Unit

Carol R. Bennett

T his section outlines the special considerations for the newborn that must undergo surgical procedures during their stay in the Neonatal Intensive Care Unit (NICU). Neonatal nurses work in the NICU and care for newborn infants born with problems including prematurity, birth defects, infection, cardiac malformations, and surgical conditions.

Caring for an infant with a surgical condition requires an extensive knowledge of newborn physiology and training to recognize and respond to complications. Neonatal nurses provide expert care for the newborn while also supporting the family. Neonatal nurses are also responsible for providing treatment that reduces pain from surgery, which is vital in the care for newborns and recovery after surgery. This requires neonatal nurses to always be reviewing current pain prevention and treatment methods.

Reducing Pain from Surgery

Pain prevention provided by the hospital is an expectation from parents. Newborns requiring intensive care undergo an average of two to ten painful experiences per day. It is not always possible to completely eliminate pain, but much is done to minimize the amount and intensity of pain. In the NICU, nurses are experts in providing optimal pain management, which can be especially difficult when caring for the newborn. It is difficult as newborns are in the pre-verbal stage, which lasts from 0-12 months. Because newborns cannot self-report pain, nurses are trained using dedicated pain-assessment tools or scales which observe the newborn's physiologic state and behavioral patterns.

Nurses will observe for changes in the newborn's heart rate, breathing rate, blood pressure, oxygen content in the blood, and changes in behavior such as crying, facial expressions, and body movements. Narcotics, such as morphine and fentanyl, provide for pain control after surgery. Morphine remains the standard in the NICU. Other medications, dexmedetomidine and acetaminophen, are also used postoperatively. An intravenous (IV) catheter is most often in place and these medications are delivered through the IV.

A team approach, which involves including the parents of the newborn, is especially important for pain prevention. Additional ways for parents to help effectively reduce pain in their newborn include; oral sucrose (sugar water), breastfeeding, pacifier use, kangaroo care (skin-to-skin contact with parent), stroking, rocking, swaddling, and limiting loud noises and bright lights. Parents, nurses, pharmacists, and the medical team can work together to reduce a newborn's pain from surgery.

Common Types of Newborn Surgery

Some of the most common types of surgery performed on newborns are stomach and/or intestinal, heart, urinary, and brain. Surgery to relieve intestinal obstruction is very common after birth. Newborns with intestinal obstructions are a major cause for surgery in all pediatric hospitals and almost always present at birth.

Newborns who are close to term should pass a meconium stool within the first day of life. Any delay in the passage of meconium stool beyond 24 hours raises concern among neonatal nurses. A distended and tense abdomen, vomiting, and sensitivity to handling and movement are characteristics among newborns born with an intestinal obstruction. Surgical newborns receive the highest priority, when presenting with symptoms of intestinal obstruction. The earlier the obstruction is detected the better the outcome is for the baby.

Challenges and Difficulties

There are challenges and difficulties when a surgical newborn presents in the NICU. Most babies cannot be fed immediately and require an IV. Keeping the newborn without nutrition by mouth requires an IV containing intravenous fluids. Ideally, surgical babies have a central venous catheter in place after surgery for multiple drug infusions and intravenous nutrition. Central venous catheters include; umbilical catheters, a peripherally inserted central catheter (PICC), and for more medium or long-term use, a tunneled catheter called a "Broviac". After major surgery nurses are responsible for accurate fluid management. In addition to fluid management, temperature regulation is fundamental to newborn care.

Temperature control

Newborns are particularly likely to become cold. Their skin is thin and permeable (porous) enabling them to lose heat easily as they have very little fat for insulation. They also have little ability to generate heat on their own. Unlike older children who shiver when they're cold as a way to create heat, newborns are unable to shiver and thus it is important to keep newborns warm. In term infants, skin temperature is maintained at 37 degrees Celsius (98.6 degrees Fahrenheit). In the NICU, newborns are placed in an isolette (incubator) or under a radiant warmer to help maintain their temperature. An isolette provides a constant warm environment even when the doors are opened. Temperatures are monitored closely before, during, and after surgery to prevent heat loss. After surgery, the nurse helps parents to focus on their baby rather than the surrounding intensive care area. Even in the immediate postoperative period a parent can take the baby's temperature, sit quietly at the bedside and hold their baby's hand. Early involvement in caregiving helps parents to feel more included in their baby's recovery. Mothers are encouraged to express breast milk and often benefit from seeing a lactation consultant.

Breastfeeding

Feeding issues can cause a barrier to a mother's confidence and mother-baby interaction especially when it comes to breastfeeding. Because of separation stress and overall concern for the baby's well-being, mothers of surgical newborns have more difficulty in establishing breastfeeding. It is important for the mother to know that breast milk is the best choice and that she is involved in the decisions regarding the feeding of her baby. When the baby returns from surgery, feeding is usually started as soon as possible, but this can often depend on the type of surgery and the response of the baby. Small feeds of breast milk given every three hours can help in the earlier feeding of newborns that have undergone surgery. Breast milk has an important immunologic value for the surgical newborn and protects them against infections.

Preventing Infection

The newborn is susceptible to infection following surgery. The most effective way to handle surgical infectious complications is to stop them from occurring. To prevent infection, nurses provide strict and careful hand washing and wound care. They also monitor the wound site for poor healing or wound infection. The use of drains are sometimes needed after surgical procedures to help in the collection of blood and drainage from the wound. These drains are always removed as soon as possible after surgery so as to prevent infection. Antibiotics to fight infection are administered based on age and weight of the baby. Antibiotic coverage to help prevent infection is discussed with the parents when indicated.

Parents and the NICU

Being a parent of a newborn baby who requires hospitalization and surgical intervention can be very stressful. It is difficult to watch your baby undergo painful procedures. Feelings of anxiety and depression are common and sometimes last long after the baby goes home. In the postoperative period, parents are given guidance and encouraged to participate in their newborn's care to the extent that is comfortable for them. Parent participation helps to alleviate anxiety and has great influence on the baby recovering from surgery.

Before taking your baby home, you should be able to answer "YES" to all of the following statements:

✓ I know when to call 911.

✓ I know the names, dosages and directions for giving ALL medications that have been prescribed for my child.

✓ I have prescriptions for all the medications that have been prescribed for my baby.

✓ I have a thermometer, and I know how to take my baby's temperature.

✓ I know that I should call my baby's pediatrician if my baby appears to be in pain, has a fever or is not wetting diapers.

✓ I know how to use the monitoring equipment that may be sent home with my baby.

✓ I know how to put my baby to bed in a crib to be safe.

✓ I know how to place my baby in her car seat.

✓ I know how to position my baby to minimize breathing difficulties.

✓ I know how to protect my baby from an infection.

✓ I know when my baby's follow-up appointments are scheduled, or I know how to schedule my child's follow-up appointments.

✓ I have received a referral to a social worker or case manager if I have financial or social concerns that will prevent me from obtaining medications or services needed for my child's follow-up care

Are there INTERNET resources where I can learn more about premature babies and the NICU?

American Academy of Pediatrics
www.healthychildren.org

Centers for Disease Control and Prevention, Life Stages and
Populations http://www.cdc.gov/features/lifestages.html

March of Dimes
www.marchofdimes.org

Pebbles of Hope
www.pebblesofhope.org

Pediatrics

Carla Anderson & Jane Hartman

When a child is admitted to the hospital it can be a stressful event for the entire family. This chapter is intended to help you cope with and be an advocate for your child during his or her stay in the hospital.

What can I expect to happen during the admission process?

Once you enter the hospital, you will encounter many health professionals. Do not be alarmed if several different caregivers come into your child's room during the admission process. While the doctor may be asking questions, members of the nursing staff may be performing a physical assessment and obtaining important vital signs, such as a blood pressure and temperature.

You may be asked many questions about your child. The history that you provide is very important in planning the care of your child. It may seem irrelevant and time-consuming, but please be as accurate as possible during this interview. You will be asked about the birth of your child and any other hospitalizations. Your child's allergies, immunization status and exposure to other people with illness, including recent travel outside of the United States, are all important information.

How will my child be kept safe during his or her hospitalization?

First and foremost, everyone of your child's caregivers are committed to keeping your child safe. Many children's hospitals have restricted access for visitors and staff. This restriction may include requiring visitors to check in and obtain a guest pass before entering the nursing unit. You may also notice that a badge or swipe card is required to access specific areas. A "safe word" is commonly required if someone is calling in to inquire about your child. You will be asked to choose your safe word when your child is admitted. If you have concerns about security or need to change your safe word during your child's hospital stay, please tell your nurse.

In many children's hospitals the staff may be identified by their specific uniforms and also must wear a photo identification badge. If you are unsure about the staff caring for your child, please do not hesitate to ask them their name, title and role in your child's care.

How can I stay involved in the care of my child?

An extremely important thing to remember is that you are the expert when it comes to your child. You know him or her better than anyone, and while your child is in the hospital you will become an important part of his or her caregiving team. Most hospitals allow parents or guardians to visit around the clock.

At least once a day your caregiving team will "round" on your child. During this time your child will be examined by members of the caregiving team and his or her plan of care will be reviewed and shared with you.

You are encouraged to:

- Ask questions: There is no such thing as a "dumb" question when it comes to your child. It is not uncommon for healthcare staff to use medical terms which you may not understand. Ask for an explanation of these medical terms. If the explanation is still unclear, ask if one of the team members can return after rounds to provide clarification and further explanation.
- Be an active participant in your child's rounds. Many children's hospitals have "family-centered rounds," where parents are an integral part of the team.
- Express your hopes for your child's progress each day.
- Ask your child's physician about the daily goals/plan for your child.
- Share your hopes and goals for your child upon discharge. Discharge planning should be a topic each day your child is in the hospital. Indicate what you feel may be most helpful in order to care for your child at home.

If, at any time, you feel that something is "not quite right" with your child, please voice your concerns to the nurse immediately. You may be the first person to recognize the subtle signs that your child is getting worse.

If you feel your concerns are not being addressed, you are encouraged to activate a medical emergency team, sometimes called a Rapid Response Team, via phone. The medical emergency team is made up of caregivers who will come and assess your child urgently. Parents may activate a medical emergency team. You will be provided with the contact information of the medical emergency team when your child is admitted.

How should I keep track of what happens during my child's hospitalization?

You and your child may meet many different caregivers during a stay in the hospital. Keeping each person's role straight can be quite confusing. It is a good idea to request business cards from your child's doctors and other healthcare professionals. Note the specialty, if appropriate, and the date and purpose of his or her visit, on the back of the card. Be sure to write down any questions you would like to ask them during their next visit. You may also wish to start a daily diary in a notebook or binder and keep it with you at all times. A blank calendar can be helpful to keep track of small milestones or accomplishments that may happen during a long hospital stay. You can collect all of the business cards you are given in a clear plastic sandwich bag.

What services are available to me, my family or my close friends while my child is in the hospital?

In order for you to care for your child, it is very important for you to care for yourself. There are several hospital services that may be of benefit to you. Family room or lodging arrangements, such as Ronald McDonald House, provide a place for you to take a break and rest, access a computer, shower, wash clothes, eat/snack and exercise. Many hospitals offer additional services or assistance provided through volunteers, child life specialists, social workers or spiritual care providers. These services are often available for the whole family, not just the child who is hospitalized.

If you have a specific need or medical condition, please tell your nurse. These might include diabetes, pregnancy or heart conditions.

Why might my child need to stay in the pediatric intensive care unit (PICU)?

There are times when your child's condition may require frequent monitoring or assessment. If this is the case, he or she may be admitted to the pediatric intensive care unit (PICU). The caregivers in this ICU have specialized pediatric critical care training which enables them to care for seriously ill children.

Whether the PICU hospitalization was anticipated or not, you may feel a wide range of emotions and physical symptoms such as numbness, fear, heart-racing, loss of control, stomach aches, unquenchable thirst or lack of appetite. This is normal and expected.

When your child arrives to the PICU, you may be asked to remain in the waiting room to allow the medical team to evaluate and start treatment. After your child's vital signs (heart rate, breathing and blood pressure) are stable, you will be brought into the room. Here are some things you may find in this PICU:

- Frequent monitoring of vital signs
- Additional equipment, such as breathing machines and specialized medication pumps
- Multiple IV lines and tubes coming out of your child
- Frequent beeping of monitors

Your child's nurse will provide frequent examinations and interventions. He or she will likely remain near your child's bed or just outside their room for most of the day. The PICU doctors and other caregivers will round multiple times during the day. You are invited to be part of the discussion. While parents may stay at the bedside around the clock, there will be times when you will be asked to briefly step out in order for the staff to do a specific task.

What do I need to know before my child is discharged?

Before your child is discharged your nurse will review written discharge instructions, line by line. If there is something that you do not understand, stop the nurse and ask him or her to explain.

Please pay particular attention to your child's discharge medications. Make sure that all the medications that your child was taking at home prior to being admitted are reviewed and either renewed or stopped. Also, you will be asked to read back the list of medications and describe why your child is taking each one. If the medication is a special one that can only be obtained at the hospital, make sure that this is filled prior to leaving the hospital.

Sometimes children are sent home from the hospital with special pieces of equipment or special intravenous devices (IVs). You should feel comfortable in caring for your child in regard to this equipment. If you are not comfortable, please advise your nurse so further education can be done prior to discharge.

A home healthcare agency nurse may come to your home to help you care for your child. If this is the case, make sure all of your questions are answered prior to discharge. You will need to know when to expect the nurse to arrive, how to contact the nurse or the agency and what care the nurse will provide.

Before taking your child home, you should be able to answer "YES" to all of the following statements:

✓ I know when to call 911.

✓ I know the names, dosages and directions for giving ALL medications that have been prescribed for my child.

✓ I have prescriptions for all the medications that have been prescribed for my child.

✓ I have the contact information of the physician who will oversee my child's care after they leave the hospital.

✓ I know when my child's follow-up appointments are scheduled, or I know how to schedule my child's follow-up appointments.

✓ I have received a referral to a social worker or case manager if I have financial or social concerns that will prevent me from obtaining medications or services needed for my child's follow-up care.

Are there INTERNET resources where I can learn more about health resources for the children?

The American Academy of Pediatrics' Health Children website
www.healthychildren.org

Kidshealth
www.kidshealth.org

Individuals with Special Needs

Jane Hartman & Erica Yates

Hospitalization is a stressful time for anyone. This can be especially difficult for your family member who has sight impairment, hearing impairment, developmental issues, or mental health issues . It can also be stressful for family members or significant others. This chapter will help those with special needs and their families to navigate their hospital stay.

How do I communicate my loved one's needs to his or her caregiving team?

One of the most important roles that the nurse fulfills is to be an advocate for their patients. This means that the nurse acts in their patients' best interests and anticipates their needs. Nurses can best advocate when they are aware of their patients' needs, wishes and preferences.

During the admission process and throughout the hospital stay, it is very important that you or your loved one's special needs and preferences be addressed. In order to make the hospitalization experience as pleasant as possible, anything that would help ease the stress and anxiety of the hospital stay should be discussed with the nurse. Please let the nurse know if you are available via phone for any questions when you are not at the hospital.

- Consider discussing all of the following with your nurse:
- Specific routines: activities, time schedules, exercises, television shows, etc.
- The best way to communicate with your loved one
- Assistive devices such as canes
- Security Items: blankets, stuffed animals, clothing, etc.
- Music
- Bedding and sleep routine
- Diet/feeding: foods, special utensils, feeding routines or schedules
- Positioning: what is most comfortable for the patient
- Medication administration: times, routines
- Special wheelchairs, seats or apparatus and how they work
- Bathing preferences
- Whether your loved one uses an assistive or service animal at home. Many hospitals allow an assistive or service animal to stay with their owner provided the animal receives proper feeding and exercise.

What questions might caregivers ask about my loved one?

The nurse and other caregivers may ask any of the following questions to better understand how to provide the best care for your loved one:

- Describe what a typical day at home would include.
- How may I best communicate with your loved one?
- How may I assist your loved one with getting up and around?
- How may I approach your loved one so as not to startle them when I enter the room?

- How does your loved one best deal with painful procedures? (For example: IV starts, blood draws.)
- What helps to calm your loved one? (For example: music, holding hand, stroking forehead.)
- What types of activities does your loved one enjoy? (For example: music, TV, movies, crafts.)
- What are some specific dislikes, or what might make your loved one anxious? (For example: loud noises or crying babies.)

How will caregivers work with my loved one?

Once the nursing staff is aware of your loved one's needs, they will be able to form an individualized plan of care. The nursing staff will do their best to provide the same type of care that the patient receives at home. However, this may not always be possible due to things such as time constraints, testing schedules and variation in supplies.

If your loved one finds the change in routine upsetting, caregivers will make every effort to calm them using strategies that were identified during the admission process. At times the use of medication may be considered if they are posing a threat to themselves or others.

Bedside caregivers may provide your loved one with a special call light or other adaptive equipment. Your loved one should always have a way to call for their nursing caregiver within reach.

The nursing staff will use the information provided to form a relationship with your loved one. When possible, the same nurses will be assigned to care for the same patients. This is called continuity of care and is helpful in forming nurse-patient relationships. The family is very important in initiating a trusting relationship with the staff. When you feel comfortable, your loved one will feel comfortable as well.

What suggestions do you have to make the hospital stay go smoothly?

- Bring in an updated list of medications and telephone numbers of physicians who provide care. You may want to keep these lists on a computer file for ease in updating.
- Bring in any security items that will help your loved one.
- Start a binder with dividers on the health history of your loved one. A quick summary of doctor visits, hospitalizations, immunizations, etc. in a file can help keep the health history straight.
- Stay with your loved one, if possible. While we encourage families to stay with their loved ones in the hospital, we are aware that you may need a break or are unable to due to other commitments. Please let us know as much as possible about any special techniques or routines you use to help your loved one prior to leaving.
- Ask if your loved one may wear his or her own clothing instead of a hospital gown.
- Take a tour of the hospital, including the areas that they may go for tests, procedures, etc.
- Ensure that your loved one has been provided with a tour of their room. If they are sight impaired, the furniture or supplies in the room may be moved to allow them to move around safely.
- Encourage your loved one to touch, smell, hear, see and taste anything that he/she will experience during their stay.
- Ask caregivers to allow your loved one to "play" with medical equipment that they plan to use. For instance, touching a surgical mask, gloves, bandages, intravenous tubing or syringes without needles may help them become more familiar with the items that caregivers will be using and may ease your loved ones' fear of the unknown.
- Let your loved one's caregivers know if he or she appears to be nervous, uncomfortable or in pain. They may not recognize your

loved ones' cues. Healing occurs much quicker when the patient is comfortable and not in pain.

How should I prepare for discharge from the hospital?

As your loved one's condition changes, they may be moved to a different level of care. This can be particularly stressful as they may get used to the environment in one setting and then be moved to another. When care is transitioned to new caregivers, whether physicians or nurses, handoff communication is given.

Handoff communication is sometimes referred to as "report". You may be asked to be involved in this handoff communication to ensure that you understand the plan of care. This is a great opportunity for you meet new caregivers, ask questions and clarify things about the patient's plan of care. You may have suggestions on how to ease this transition, and nurses welcome this information.

Before going home, you should be able to answer "YES" to all of the following statements:

✓ I know when to call 911.

✓ I know the names, dosages and directions for giving ALL medications that have been prescribed for my loved one.

✓ I know sign and symptoms of my loved one's worsening condition and whom to call.

Geriatrics

Julie Simon, Anne Vanderbilt & Karen Distelhorst

This chapter is written both for the patient who may be an "older adult" and for the caregiver who may be caring for an older adult. Adults aged 65 years and older make up about 13% of the total population in the United States. As the "baby boom" generation ages and people live longer, even more of our population will be considered "older adults." Most older adults will have at least one chronic illness.

One of the fastest growing groups is the "older old," people who are 75 years or older. Hospitalization can pose even more of a challenge for this group, especially with the changing environment of healthcare. Changes in payment systems and regulations are rapidly transforming healthcare. There was a time where hospital stays were longer, but today we know that it is best to keep hospital days to a minimum to reduce the chance of complications.

Why should I, as an older adult, try to stay out of the hospital?

For older adults, any hospitalization is a threat to independence. Hospital-acquired infections, functional decline, delirium and pressure ulcers are just a few of the things that can come with a longer hospitalization. Functional decline begins as soon as 24 hours of being bedridden, so early ambulation is very important. Older adults also take longer to recover strength and functioning after a hospitalization and may need physical therapy to return to previous level of functioning.

The key to staying as independent as possible is to do as much for yourself as possible (or allow the older adult you are caring for to do as much as they are able). Also, you need to stay long enough to get appropriate treatment, but prepare for the earliest possible discharge by sharing any information or decisions that may affect your discharge with caregivers as soon as possible. This way you are not in the hospital longer than needed. Discharge planning should begin the day of admission in order to keep your stay as short and efficient as possible.

How long should I expect to be in the hospital?

Older adults have longer hospital stays and are more at risk for readmissions than younger patients. The average length of stay for someone 65 years or older is 5.5 days. If a patient falls or develops a hospital-acquired infection, this can be even longer. Your nurses will develop a plan of care to protect your safety by preventing falls and infections.

How do I talk to my nurse or my family member's nurse?

Be honest: Do not be embarrassed to say you do not understand or if you are having a hard time hearing instructions or seeing papers that you need to sign. Your nurses need to know if you usually have a hearing aid or glasses.

Ask Questions: It is OK to ask if you do not understand something. Some older adults are used to a system of medicine where "the doctor knows best" and is not to be questioned. Doctors and nurses today know that patient participation in their care is best for good outcomes. So go ahead and ask questions! If you don't get the answers you need or don't understand, keep asking.

What should I tell my nurse or my family member's nurse?

As people age, daily routines such as sleep patterns, meal times and medication schedules become increasingly important. All of us like our routines but when you are in the hospital, most of those routines are turned upside down. This can lead to confusion, nutrition problems and fatigue. Family members can be helpful here, especially if an older adult has any type of memory loss or delirium. Maintaining routine is very important to prevent or minimize confusion in the hospital. Providing information to the nurses regarding any special care routines can be very helpful. The following are examples of daily routine information that will be helpful for caregivers to know:

- Normal bedtime and any routines that help you fall asleep
- Number of meals eaten per day and any food preferences
- Gender preferences of caregivers (Adherence to these preferences may not always be possible, but staff can try.)
- Activities that are part of the daily routine (watching the news, reading the paper, listening to music, etc.)
- Things that help you relax or feel more comfortable
- Bathing habits or preferences

The nurses and staff look so busy; what do I do if I need something?

The nurses are here for YOU. You are not a bother to the caregiving staff. Some older adults are hesitant to ask for help or use the call light because the nurses are "so busy." Using your call light is one of the most important ways to reduce your likelihood of falling. Your caregivers should check on you regularly. (This is called "purposeful hourly rounding.") When they come in, ask for help. It may also be helpful to write down questions you would like to ask your nurse or doctor so you can remember to ask when they are available. (Only wait to ask questions that don't need immediate attention.) This way you don't feel like you keep calling for the nurse. However, even if you do forget a question, please still call!

What should I look for in a hospital for an older adult?

Check for hospitals with quality and NICHE initiatives. NICHE stands for Nurses Improving Care for Healthsystem Elders. It is a designation for hospitals that pay extra attention to the specialized needs of older adult patients. NICHE helps emphasize patients' and families' needs and improve patient outcomes. NICHE facilities generally value the older adult and practice a lot of collaboration between doctors, nurses and other supportive staff (social workers, physical therapy, pharmacy, etc.).

Another term that often signals specialized care for older adults is an ACE (Acute Care of the Elderly) unit. Nurses on ACE units have received specialized training, and the patients who are admitted are generally all older adults or meet certain other criteria. Often there have been environmental changes to enhance the comfort and care of older adults.

Though it may sound counterintuitive, many times providing good care for older adults means staying in the hospital for the shortest time possible. The longer an older adult is hospitalized, the more likely the patient is to experience complications. Also, many interventions are best kept in place for the shortest time possible or avoided altogether. For example, a urinary catheter or heart monitor has its place in treatment, but is best used for a short time or not at all, if it can be helped.

What happens to older adults when they get admitted to the hospital?

Older adults are at risk for several "geriatric syndromes" that may occur when in the hospital. Listed below are the most common syndromes.

- **Delirium**: Delirium is a sudden change in mental status or sudden confusion that develops over hours to days. Delirium affects 10 to 30% of patients in the hospital and more than 50% of people in high-risk populations, such as the intensive care unit. If you notice any change in your loved one's behavior, even if it is minor, please bring it to the nurse's attention right away. Nurses routinely screen patients to detect subtle delirium and are skilled in interventions to minimize confusion. Family members can help by creating a calm and reassuring environment. It is important for the patient to have their hearing aids, glasses and adequate hydration and walking to prevent or help reduce delirium

- **Sleep disturbance**: Hospital-related sleep problems are common in older adults. Very often patients report they cannot fall asleep or stay asleep while they are in the unfamiliar hospital environment. It is best to promote sleep with relaxation techniques such as a back rub, warm beverage or music. Sleeping medication should only be used in low doses for the shortest period of time due to the high possibility of side effects in older adults.

- **Eating problems**: Older adults are more prone to weight loss and appetite problems while hospitalized. Restrictive diets, long periods of time without food due to tests and lack of assistance can all lead to malnutrition. Family members can help the older adult by reviewing the menu with them and selecting appropriate meals, bringing appropriate snacks and staying with patients during meals. It is essential to have dentures or other devices needed at meals times.

- **Urinary incontinence**: It is very common in hospitals for older adults to have difficulty getting to the bathroom for their toileting needs, which may cause urinary incontinence or accidents. Also, indwelling urinary catheters (called Foleys) are frequently needed for a short time due to medical or surgical conditions, increasing the risk of urinary tract infections. Patients should go to the bathroom frequently with the assistance of nursing staff as needed. Patients should drink adequate fluid to prevent dehydration and urine retention. Patients and family members should also be assertive in asking that Foley catheters be removed as soon as possible.

- **Skin breakdown**: Older adults are at a greater risk for developing skin breakdown while hospitalized. (See chapter on Preventing Pressure Ulcers.)
- **Falls**: Older adults are at a greater risk having a fall while hospitalized. (See chapter on Preventing Falls.)

Older adults tend to display symptoms of illness differently than younger adults. For instance, with infection there may not be a fever but instead, a change in mental status. For caregivers of older adults, always call the provider if there is a sudden onset of confusion or rapid decline in the patient's ability to care for themselves. Even if there are existing memory problems, a sudden change can indicate a serious medical condition.

As a family member or caregiver, how can I help?

There are three primary ways to help your loved one:

Advocate: Older adults need an advocate when they are in the hospital, someone who is knowledgeable of the home situation and the older adult's wishes related to healthcare. Selecting a family spokesperson is highly recommended. A spokesperson is good for anyone in the hospital. There is a lot of information to take in; it's always good to have an extra set of eyes and ears.

Ideally, in a planned admission the patient should identify an assertive person to serve as an advocate. This should be an individual with good communication skills. Sometimes different family members bring different skills – one may be good with finances, one with planning, one with physical care, etc. Families that work together find it less stressful to advocate for their older adult member.

Communicate: In most cases, family members cannot be with the older adult around the clock in the hospital. Use a communication notebook or log to leave hospital caregivers important information about your older adult family member. Ask your nurse when the physician/providers "round" so family members can be present. Having another person present when the doctor sees the patient is helpful in remembering key information. If someone cannot be there, write down questions for the doctor and have the nurse assist you with obtaining the information.

Supervise: Sometimes, when older adults are extremely confused (called delirium), family may be asked to help with supervision, if they are able. This is not because the hospital cannot provide staff, but because a familiar face and presence can help minimize some of the effects of delirium. Your nurse can help teach you ways to deal with confusion, such as distraction or re-orientation. But you are not alone! Your nurses and patient care assistants are there to provide for care and safety.

What should I expect when leaving the hospital?

Being in the hospital can really take a toll on your strength. You should expect to require a little time to get back to your previous level of activity and independence. The amount of help that you will need depends on your strength and endurance, as well as the physical layout of your home environment. For example, if you live in a two-story home and the bathroom is upstairs, you may need to do some planning. Your hospital should provide assistance with discharge planning, either from a registered nurse or a social worker.

You may require assistive equipment when you are discharged, including the following:

- **Walking aids**: You may need a cane or walker, even temporarily, to help you ambulate safely while your strength returns.
- **Bathroom equipment**: Consider if you can get to the bathroom or if you can bathe safely. Items to consider are a portable commode (which can double as a raised toilet seat), shower chair, railings or a hand-held shower.
- **Safety**: Make sure that you have access to a portable phone or mobile device. Some older adults are at a high risk for falling at home. A personal emergency response system, also known as a medical alert unit, may be a good idea. This is a wireless button worn around the wrist or as necklace that allows an older adult to call for help in an emergency.

If I can't go home alone after the hospital, what help is available or where else might I go?

There are several home care and residential care options if you or your loved one need assistance. They include the following:

- **Home Healthcare**: Most older adults prefer to remain in their own home when recovering from an illness. For qualifying homebound patients, skilled home care can provide services such as nursing, personal care aid, social work and therapy, for a brief period of time while you recover from an illness. Skilled home care is paid for by your health insurance.
- **Non-skilled home care**: Often times after skilled home care has ended, older adults may need some additional assistance in basic activities of daily living, such as bathing or meal preparation. These non-skilled services may be provided by family members or non-skilled home care agencies. These services are paid for privately or through long-term care insurance. Depending on your income you may qualify for Medicaid and/or special state run programs to provide basic care in your home. One such program is

Passport. You can contact your local Area Agency on Aging to find out about programs to help you remain at home. You can find your local agency through the Administration on Aging website (www. aoa.gov).

- **Long-Term Acute Care** (LTAC): This is a type of specialty-hospital for patients with serious medical problems that require intense nursing care for a long period of time.
- Skilled Nursing or Rehabilitation Facilities (SNF): Sometimes older adults become too weak to immediately return home, or they need ongoing treatment. A short term stay for nursing or physical therapy may be needed.
- **Assisted Living**: This is an ongoing living arrangement for people who need help with multiple activities of daily living.
- **Long-Term Care Facilities** (Nursing Home): This option is for those people who will not be able to return to independent living.

How do I avoid coming back to the hospital?

The best way to prevent being readmitted to the hospital is to make sure you are ready to leave the first time. Most hospitals have a specially-trained nurse or social worker called a discharge planner or case manager who can help you plan for your home going needs.

Before going home, you should be able to answer "YES" to all of the following statements:

✓ My pain is under good control, and I have a clear plan how to manage my pain if it increases

✓ I have prescriptions if pain medication is indicated.

✓ I know what medications I should take at home.

✓ I have the supplies I will need at home, such as walkers, oxygen, a hospital bed, etc.

✓ I understand what symptoms require attention.

✓ I understand how to perform tasks that I will need to do at home, such as how to change my dressing, give myself a shot, manage a tube feeding as needed, etc.

✓ I know who and how to contact someone if needed.

✓ I know under what circumstances to call my home care nurse or primary care provider.

✓ I know when to call 911 or go to the emergency department.

✓ I have follow-up plans scheduled.

✓ I know when my home care nurse is coming or when my follow-up appointment with my primary care provider is scheduled.

Are there INTERNET resources where I can learn more about healthcare for the older adult?

American Association of Retired Persons
www.AARP.org

National Institute on Aging
www.nih.gov/nia

Nurses Improving Care for Healthsystem Elders (NICHE) Program
www.nicheprogram.org

Conclusion

Mary Beth Modic and Christina Canfield

This book has been a labor love. It was written by expert nurses who are committed to alleviating suffering, preventing complications and promoting healing in their patients. A great deal of space has been dedicated to describing the role of the bedside nurse and the impact this dedicated caregiver has not only on your hospital experience, but on your overall health as well.

Nurses have been consistently rated as the most trusted professionals in America by the Gallup Annual Poll, a position they have held every year since 1999, except 2001, when fire fighters were awarded the honor. While nurses are held in high regard by the public, most would find it difficult to describe what nurses actually do. Our hope is that this book has provided you, the reader, with invaluable information on how your nurse advocates for you, cares for you and keeps you safe.

Hospitals can be scary places. This book contains recommendations on how to have you or your loved one's needs met. The overarching theme is communication – how it is provided to you and your loved ones and how your questions, concerns and challenges are heard by members of the care-giving team. The messages in this book are summarized below:

Acknowledge the need for help. Use your call light. Patients often worry that they are being a "bother" to their nurse, so they try and get out of bed by themselves. Your nurse and nursing assistant are here to assist you so you do not fall or injure yourself.

Activate the Rapid Response Team (RRT) if you, or one of your loved ones, think that your condition is deteriorating or that something is "not right" and your symptoms are not being heard or acknowledged by your nurses and doctors.

Appreciate that you are the most important member of the caregiving team.

Ask your caregivers to introduce themselves to you and their role in your care.

Ask for additional explanations. If the reason for a test or procedure is not clear to you, ask for another explanation.

Ask for time to learn. It takes time to take in and understand all the infor-mation and teaching that is being given. Ask your nurses and doctors for time to practice giving an injection or changing a dressing. Ask for explanations in layman's terms if the instructions contain a lot of medical language.

Ask your caregivers to sit down when they are explaining or teaching you about a medication, test or procedure. This helps to enhance communica-tion as your doctor or nurse is at your eye level.

Be curious. The more that you can partner with your caregivers and actively participate, the greater understanding you will have about your plan of care.

Be honest. Tell your caregivers if you are not going to fill your prescription or have not been taking your medications as prescribed. This can help prevent complications. Perhaps another medication may be prescribed

Describe your expectations to your caregivers. This is often where communication breaks down. Sometimes patients and their loved ones have expectations that cannot be met because of the acuity of the illness or limitations of treatment options.

Express your fears and worries. Often telling your nurse, doctor or physical therapist your concerns can reduce the emotional burden you are carrying.

Find out about your plan for discharge early in your hospital stay. This will allow you to share obstacles that may prevent you from going home as planned.

Identify a family spokesperson. This will help your caregivers know the person you prefer to learn about your progress and plan of care.

Make your needs known. Share any change in your physical condition with your caregiver right away. This will allow your nurse and doctor to address the problem right away before any symptom gets worse. Some examples of a change in condition include a sudden increase in pain, difficulty breathing or an inability to urinate.

Report your dissatisfaction with your care to the nurse manager of the nursing unit or your attending doctor so that it can be resolved quickly. No one wants you to be distressed or disappointed as you are recovering from your illness.

Request another doctor if you think that your concerns, questions or complaints are not acknowledged.

SPEAK UP. All of your caregivers, but most especially your nurses and doctors want you to question and challenge us if there are differences in the information that has been provided, explanations that have been given or promises that have been made.

The best teachers are you, our patients. You teach us about hope and courage and gratitude. You remind us to slow down, take time to listen and empathize with your suffering. When we listen to you, we learn. Your voice reminds us of our purpose ... healing.

Personal Care Plan

This document can be used to record the names of all your caregivers. You can use it as journal of your care while you recover in the hospital. It can also help remind you of the tests, procedures or consults that must be completed before you are discharged.

Admission Date: _____   Anticipated Discharge Date: _____

Names of my Doctors, Physician Assistants and Nurse Practitioners:

_____

_____

_____

_____

_____

Names of my Nurses:

_____

_____

_____

_____

_____

Names of other caregivers (Dietician, Pharmacist, therapist(s)):

_____

_____

_____

Name of my Social Worker or Case Manager:

_____

_____

Name and date of scheduled tests or procedures:

_____

_____

_____

_____

What's New: Daily Update:

_____

_____

_____

_____

_____

_____

What needs to be done before I can be discharged:

_____

_____

_____

_____

Questions I still have:

_____

_____

_____

_____

Contributing Authors

Nancy M. Albert, PhD, APRN, CCNS, CHFN, CCRN, NE-BC, FAHA, FCCM, FHFSA, FAAN

Associate Chief Nursing Officer, Nursing Research and Innovation-Cleveland Clinic Health System;

Clinical Nurse Specialist, Heart Failure-Cleveland Clinic main campus

Nancy M. Albert is associate chief nursing officer for Cleveland Clinic's Office of Nursing Research and Innovation, and a clinical nurse specialist in heart failure where she uses research results in heart failure-related critical care and cardiac telemetry programs to promote evidence-based practice, patient safety and quality outcomes. Albert is also an adjunct associate professor at Case Western Reserve University, Bolton School of Nursing, Cleveland, Ohio, and a full professor at Aalborg University, Aalborg, Denmark She is the first past president of the American Association of Heart Failure Nurses, and volunteers on national committees for multiple medical, nursing, and health care organizations.

Carla Q. Anderson, MSN, APRN, CPN

Clinical Nurse Specialist, Pediatric Intensive Care Unit

Carla Q. Anderson is a clinical nurse specialist in pediatrics at Cleveland Clinic Children's. A certified pediatric nurse (CPN), Anderson has specialized in the care of the pediatric patient population since she started her career. She has worked at the five children's hospitals throughout the Midwest.

Carol R. Bennett, MSN, MBA, APRN, PCNS-BC

Clinical Nurse Specialist, Neonatal Intensive Care Unit

Carol R. Bennett is a board-certified pediatric clinical nurse specialist at Cleveland Clinic Children's. Bennett has spent over two decades caring for the pediatric patient population. Her experience includes pediatric and neonatal intensive care settings and pediatric clinical research coordination. With a personal mission to progress and continually enhance pediatric care, Bennett has initiated pediatric ethics nursing rounds, a hypothermia program and numerous quality projects in the inpatient hospital setting.

Lydia C. Booher, MSN, APRN, ACNS-BC, ONC

Advanced Practice Nurse and Physician Assistant Coordinator, Acute Pain Management Service

Lydia C. Booher is a clinical nurse specialist in orthopedics and general surgery at Cleveland Clinic main campus. With over 2 decades of experience treating patient populations throughout the globe, Booher has practiced nursing in India, Saudi Arabia and the United States. She is certified in adult health and orthopedic nursing, specializing in the care of patients undergoing total joint replacement surgeries, including those with chronic pain, spine surgeries and more. She holds special interests in Safe Patient Handling and Mobility (SPHM) programs, care of trauma patients, end-of-life care, care coordination, knee and hip arthroplasty, chronic pain and osteoporosis and is actively involved in writing and reviewing care pathways in these areas.

Christian N. Burchill, PhD, RN, CEN

Nurse Researcher, Office of Nursing Research and Innovation

Christian N. Burchill is a nurse researcher for Cleveland Clinic's Office of Nursing Research and Innovation. Dr. Burchill's program of research is in contextual and organizational factors that impact the delivery of healthcare and its outcome, and he has produced many published works on his research throughout his career. In addition to actively conducting research, Dr. Burchill mentors nurses from all professional practice arenas so that they can conduct their own rigorous research studies, disseminate their results, and translate their findings into clinical practice. He also participates in and leads interprofessional research studies and serves as a research consultant to other healthcare providers and researchers.

Christina M. Canfield, MSN, APRN, ACNS-BC, CCRN-E

Clinical Nurse Specialist, eHospital Program Manager

Christina M. Canfield is a program manager for Cleveland Clinic eHospital, the health system's homegrown ICU telemedicine program. Canfield is a board-certified adult clinical nurse specialist and critical-care registered nurse. Canfield brings a wealth of knowledge and experience to her position. In addition to medical intensive care, her expertise includes internal medicine, pulmonary, otorhinolaryngology and renal care, as well as long-term acute care.

Theresa L. Cary, MSN, APRN, ACNS-BC, CHFN, CCRN

Clinical Nurse Specialist, High Risk Patient Education

Theresa L. Cary is a board-certified adult clinical nurse specialist with a specialty in medical cardiology. One of her notable career successes includes the development of a unit-based nurse champion program designed to support staff nurses with patient care and education. Due to her success, this program has been used as a best practice throughout other inpatient units within the health system. Cary also developed an interdisciplinary heart failure patient education class that has educated more than 5,600 patients and family members in its first four years.

Stacey S. Claus, MSN, APRN, GCNS-BC, CNRN

Clinical Nurse Specialist, Magnet Program

Stacey S. Claus is a clinical nurse specialist in medical-surgical nursing at Cleveland Clinic Fairview Hospital. Throughout her career, Claus has worked to advance the professional practice of nursing and improve patient care through strategies such as quality improvement initiatives, patient fall reduction efforts and interventions to minimize hospital-acquired conditions. She is an advocate for collaboration between physicians, mid-level providers and nurses and is actively involved in ensuring successful communication within the healthcare team.

Christina M. Colvin, MSN, APRN, AOCNS

Clinical Nurse Specialist, Oncology

Christina M. Colvin is a clinical nurse specialist in Cleveland Clinic's Taussig Cancer Institute, working within the adult hematology and bone marrow transplant units as well as the Ambulatory Cancer Center. Colvin specializes in oncology, maintaining advanced oncology certification as a clinical nurse specialist (AOCNS) through the Oncology Nursing Certification Corporation. As a member of the Office of Nursing Education and Professional Practice Development, Colvin works to develop and coordinate education, safety and support initiatives for patients, their families and healthcare providers.

Jennifer P. Colwill, MSN, APRN, CCNS, PCCN

Clinical Nurse Specialist, Cardiothoracic and Thoracic Surgery

Jennifer P. Colwill is a clinical nurse specialist for Cleveland Clinic's Heart and Vascular Institute (HVI). Colwill is responsible for the oversight of all clinical practice within the cardiovascular step-down units at Cleveland Clinic's main campus. With many notable career successes, she developed a pain management nursing champion program that offers nurses a combination of education and functional tools at the bedside. Additionally, her work has significantly impacted the advancement of evidence-based practice for the prevention of catheter associated urinary tract infections. Having a career history that spans the United States, India and Saudi Arabia, Colwill began her nursing career in India after receiving her bachelor's degree from S.N.D.T. Women's University in Mumbai.

Myra A. Cook, MSN, APRN, ACNS-BC, CCRN, CSC

Clinical Nurse Specialist, Cardiovascular Intensive Care, Heart and Lung Transplant

Myra A. Cook is a board-certified adult clinical nurse specialist at Cleveland Clinic main campus. With clinical expertise in critical care, Cook's career successes include initiatives designed to reduce hospital-acquired infections and improve quality outcomes, patient safety and patient experience. Cook serves as a clinical leader in the cardiovascular intensive care units and heart and lung transplant unit. She has studied the needs of young children visiting the ICU.

Dianna Copley, MSN, APRN, ACCNS-AG, CCRN

Clinical Nurse Specialist, Internal Medicine

Dianna Copley is a board-certified adult geriatric clinical nurse specialist at Cleveland Clinic main campus. With clinical expertise in care of the critically ill adult, Copley's career successes include a publication about atrial fibrillation and collaborative work on a comprehensive sepsis care path. Copley serves as a clinical expert and resource for nurses within the medicine institute. Her interests include staff development, quality improvement and nursing research.

Tina E. Di Fiore, MSN, APRN, CNS, NNP-BC, RN

Clinical Nurse Specialist, Hillcrest Hospital Neonatal Intensive Care Unit

Tina E. DiFiore is a clinical nurse specialist for Cleveland Clinic Children's neonatal intensive care unit (NICU) at Cleveland Clinic Hillcrest Hospital. A certified neonatal nurse practitioner, DiFiore has spent the majority of her 25 years in the nursing profession caring for the neonatal patient population. She played an important role in the opening of Hillcrest Hospital's Level IIIB NICU in 2010, assisting with the design, planning and purchasing of equipment as well as education and training of all nursing staff.

Karen S. Distelhorst, MSN, APRN, RN, GCNS-BC

Clinical Nurse Specialist, Gerontology

Karen S. Distelhorst is a clinical nurse specialist in gerontology at Cleveland Clinic South Pointe Hospital. Distelhorst has spent the majority of her career caring for the geriatric patient population. In addition to her current role, Distelhorst's clinical experience includes nurse, case manager, nursing supervisor and clinical nurse specialist positions in the skilled home nursing setting, geriatric clinical nurse specialist positions at Summa Health System and The Traveling Nurse Practitioner in Akron, Ohio, and Barberton Citizen's Hospital in Barberton, Ohio.

Karen L. Guzi, MSN, APRN, ACNS-BC, BCEN

Clinical Nurse Specialist, Emergency Department

Karen L. Guzi is a board-certified adult clinical nurse specialist within Cleveland Clinic's Emergency Services Institute. With more than three decades of clinical experience, Guzi's skills and expertise consist of nurse consulting, mentoring, education and professional development, nursing research, evidence-based practice and compassionate patient care. In her current position, Guzi services Cleveland Clinic's main campus, Avon, Ohio and Twinsburg, Ohio, locations. She is a trusted resource for nursing best practices, quality monitoring and process improvement, and a mentor for all staff.

Kelly A. Haight, MSN, APRN, ACNS-BC, PCCN

Clinical Nurse Specialist, Medical Cardiology and Heart Failure

Kelly A. Haight is a board-certified adult clinical nurse specialist for the cardiovascular and thoracic step-down units at Cleveland Clinic main campus. She is an active member of various health system committees and councils, including co-chair of the Cleveland Clinic nursing pain mentor program. Haight provides educational classes to new and experienced nurses, assists in preparing staff for accreditation surveys and offers support for necessary practice changes, such as the implementation of new technology.

Jane H. Hartman, MSN, APRN, PNP-BC

Pediatric Nurse Practitioner

Jane H. Hartman is a certified pediatric nurse practitioner in the clinical nurse specialist role at Cleveland Clinic Children's. Hartman has been integral to improving patient outcomes through the dissemination of evidence-based practice, enhancements to nursing policies, protocols and procedures, collaboration with the interprofesional care team and more. She developed the Hartman Baker Pediatric Peripheral Vascular Access Algorithm which aids nurses in the decision making of starting IVs in pediatric patients.

Christina M. Henrich, MSN, RN, ACNS-BC

Clinical Nurse Specialist, Orthopedics

Christina M. Henrich is a board-certified Adult Clinical Nurse Specialist in Orthopedics at Cleveland Clinic main campus. She brings more than a decade of nursing experience to her role and has spent most of her career within the specialties of Medical-Surgical and Neuroscience nursing. Her vast clinical experience encompasses Orthopedic, Bariatric, and general surgical procedures. She is a Robert Wood Johnson Foundation Future of Nursing Scholar pursuing a doctorate in nursing concentrating on family and community care.

Kathleen M. Hill, MSN, APRN, CCNS

Clinical Nurse Specialist, Surgical Intensive Care Unit

Kathleen M. Hill is a clinical nurse specialist for the surgical intensive care unit at Cleveland Clinic's main campus. Hill is a diversified CNS, having practiced in a variety of intensive care settings, including coronary care, heart failure, cardiac surgery, and medical and surgical intensive care. She actively lectures and publishes works on critical care and advanced practice nursing, including atrial fibrillation, hemodynamic monitoring, family presence in the intensive care unit, prescriptive authority for the CNS, role delineation for advanced practice nurses.

Marianela E. Iuppa, DNP, MS, RN-BC, NEA-BC, FHIMSS

Associate Chief Nursing Officer, Office of Nursing Informatics

Marianela (Nelita) Iuppa is Cleveland Clinic's associate chief nursing officer for nursing informatics. Iuppa has been a leading figure in the Office of Nursing Informatics, devising countless automated technology solutions for clinical care including: electronic nursing documentation, web design, interoperability of systems, mobile devices, business intelligence, clinical decision support, simulation, and patient centered solutions. She is active nationally as a leader in the specialty of Nursing Informatics and Technology Innovation through her lectures, board member participation, publications, and education she provides to nurses practicing in this field.

Diana Karius MS, APRN, CNS, AOCN, CHPN

Clinical Nurse Specialist, Oncology

Diana L. Karius is a clinical nurse specialist for the oncology and palliative medicine units at Cleveland Clinic main campus. Karius is a trusted leader with over 30 years of nursing experience and certification in both oncology (AOCN) and palliative medicine (CHPN). She is responsible for education, monitoring and enhancing practice on inpatient / out-patient oncology and palliative medicine nursing units. Karius serves as a primary chemotherapy resource for the health system. Karius has served as adjunct faculty for students from Case Western, Kent State, Ursuline and Akron University. She has been the recipient of the Mary Nowotny award for excellence in cancer nursing education from the Oncology Nursing Society.

Nancy J. Kaser, MSN, BS, APRN, ACNS-BC, NEA-BC

Clinical Nurse Specialist, Internal Medicine

Nancy J. Kaser is a clinical nurse specialist in internal medicine at Cleveland Clinic main campus. Kaser has taken on many roles including staff nurse, case manager, consultant, nursing educator and director. She is an experienced caregiver and leader whose passion for nursing excellence drives her current work in the areas of mobility / safe patient handling and advocacy & health policy.

Deborah G. Klein, MSN, APRN, ACNS-BC, CCRN, CHFN, FAHA

Clinical Nurse Specialist, Coronary and Heart Failure Intensive Care Units

Deborah G. Klein is a clinical nurse specialist in the coronary and heart failure intensive care units, and cardiac accelerated recovery, cardiac short-stay and post-anesthesia care units at Cleveland Clinic main campus. Klein boasts more than three decades of experience in critical care practice, education, consultation and research, having significantly advanced the nursing profession throughout her career. She is known for her work in therapeutic hypothermia post-cardiac arrest, pain assessment in patients who are unable to communicate pain, and end-of-life care.

Kate E. Klein, MS, APRN, ANCP-BC, CCRN

Acute Care Nurse Practitioner, Neurocritical Care

Kate E. Klein is an acute care nurse practitioner practicing in the Neurological Intensive Care Unit within Cleveland Clinic's Cerebrovascular Center. Klein entered the nursing profession in an intensive care unit and focused her practice as a nurse practitioner on the care of patients critically ill with neurological injury. In addition to her clinical practice, Klein has studied and developed practice improvements aimed at optimizing patient's recovery from critical illness and clinician safety. She is a member of the American Association of Critical Care Nurses, Neurocritical Care Society and Society of Critical Care Medicine within which she actively disseminates her work.

Meredith A. Lahl, MSN, APRN, PCNS-BC, PPNP-BC, CPON

Executive Director, Associate Chief Nursing Officer Advanced Practice

Meredith A. Lahl is senior director of advanced practice nursing for the Cleveland Clinic heath system and a pediatric clinical nurse specialist at Cleveland Clinic main campus. Lahl is responsible for the oversight and supervision of the scope of practice, recruitment, quality, credentialing and privileging of Cleveland Clinic's approximately 900 advanced practice nurses. Lahl's career also includes extensive pediatric experience with a focus on the care of the child with cancer.

V. Maria Masina, MSN, APRN, AGCNS-BC

Clinical Nurse Specialist, Colorectal Surgery and Bariatrics

V. Maria Masina is a board-certified adult clinical nurse specialist at Cleveland Clinic main campus. Masina's experience consists of nurse consulting, mentoring and education, with focused efforts on evidence-based practice, professional development and nursing research. She serves as a resource for nursing staff members on topics such as nursing best practices, quality monitoring and process improvement.

Mary Beth Modic, DNP, APRN, CNS, CDE

Clinical Nurse Specialist, Diabetes

Mary Beth Modic is a Clinical Nurse Specialist in Diabetes at Cleveland Clinic in Cleveland, Ohio. She is also the Director of Interprofessional Enrichment in the Center for Excellence in Healthcare Communication at Cleveland Clinic. She is also a certified diabetes educator. She is the co-creator and facilitator of an innovative clinical leadership empowerment program for bedside nurses known as LEAD. She led the curriculum revision for the Cleveland Clinic Diabetes Self-Management Education (DSME) program which was based on extensive patient feedback. Modic's work is concentrated on providing comprehensive diabetes care using the most current research and promoting the use of empathy in communication with patients and colleagues.

Marie Namey, APRN, MSCN

Clinical Nurse Specialist, Mellen Center/Neurologic Institute

Marie Namey has been Advanced Practice Nurse at the Mellen Center for Multiple Sclerosis Treatment and Research at the Cleveland Clinic Foundation since its inception. She is responsible for assessment, treatment planning and follow-up of multiple sclerosis patients. She has specific interest on patient education and bladder, bowel management. Namey is a member of the local MS Society Chapter Healthcare Advisory Committee and the Chapter Program Committee. She also serves as a member of the Multiple Sclerosis Association of America Healthcare Advisory Committee. She has been a member of the Consortium of Multiple Sclerosis Centers since 1986 and has served as secretary, vice president and president of that organization. She currently chairs the Advocacy Committee. She is a founding member, past president and currently chairs the Scholarship Committee for the International Organization of Multiple Sclerosis Nurses.

Lynda Newman, MSN, APRN, ACNS-BC, NP-C

Nurse Practitioner, Digestive Disease Institute

Lynda N. Newman is currently a Nurse Practitioner in Gastroenterology at the Cleveland Clinic, specializing in Nutrition Support and Anemia Management. Newman's extensive experience includes development of the Home Dialysis programs (Peritoneal Dialysis (PD) and Nocturnal Home Hemodialysis) and the Chronic Kidney Disease Education and Anemia Management Clinic for University Hospitals, Case Medical Center. She has won awards for Clinical Excellence from Sigma Theta Tau, Delta Xi Chapter; the Case Western Reserve Nursing Alumni Association and the Cleveland Plain Dealer.

Shannon A. Rives, MSN, APRN, ACNS-BC, CCRN, CMSRN

Clinical Nurse Specialist, Hepatology and Transplant

Shannon A. Rives is a clinical nurse specialist with the medical-surgical telemetry, gastroenterology/hepatology and transplant special care units at Cleveland Clinic main campus. With nearly a decade of direct clinical nursing experience, Rives has concentrated her nursing career in the cardiovascular and critical care patient populations within the Cleveland Clinic health system.

Ann Roach, MSN, APRN, ACNS-BC, RNC-OB, RNC-MNN

Nurse Manager, Perinatal Nursing

Ann Roach has recently moved to the management position of Medina's Labor, Delivery, Recovery & Post-partum unit from her unique role of Perinatal Clinical Nurse Specialist. She has spoken extensively and educated continuously to various audiences from nursing students to community groups on her great love of all things obstetric related. Her current responsibilities include making Medina Hospital the best delivering hospital in the Cleveland Clinic Health care system.

Ronald A. Rock, MSN, APRN, ACNS-BC

Clinical Nurse Specialist, Nurse Manager, Wound Ostomy Continence (WOC) Nursing

Ronald A. Rock is a nurse manager for Cleveland Clinic's WOC nursing team and an Advanced Practice Clinical Nurse Specialist at Cleveland Clinic main campus. Rock is a recognized clinical expert in the use of negative pressure wound therapy to manage complex surgical and chronic wounds in both adult and pediatric patient populations. His comprehensive knowledge and innovative wound care techniques have been applied on numerous complex wounds, ranging from open chest, open abdomens, spinal and perineal wounds. He is experienced in the development of various healthcare policies, procedures and continuing education programs and is a sought-after wound therapy consultant.

Karen Schulz, MSN, APRN, ACNS-BC

Clinical Nurse Specialist, Manager Bariatric Surgery

Karen Schulz, MSN, CNS, CBN is a licensed as Advanced Practice Nurse and certified by the American Society for Metabolic and Bariatric Surgery. She has over two decades of experience in outpatient bariatric surgery. Her specialties include pre-operative surgery medical evaluation and post-operative bariatric follow up. Ms. Schulz is past president of the American Society for Metabolic and Bariatric Surgery, and serves on their executive council.

Sandy L. Siedlecki, PhD, APRN, CNS

Senior Nurse Scientist, Office of Research and Innovation

Sandra L. Siedlecki is a senior nurse scientist with the Cleveland Clinic Nursing Office of Research and Innovation. Dr. Siedlecki is actively involved in a program of research for chronic non-malignant pain syndrome patients, as well as research on the effects of complementary therapies on health outcomes. In addition, she has an ongoing interest in chronicity and its impact on patients and their caregivers. With more than two decades of didactic and clinical nursing teaching experience, Dr. Siedlecki has instructed and educated students at five colleges, universities and schools of nursing. Presently, she is an adjunct assistant professor at both Case Western Reserve University and the University of Akron.

Julie N. Simon, MSN, APRN, ACNS-B C

Clinical Nurse Specialist, Internal Medicine and Geriatrics

Julie N. Simon is a clinical nurse specialist for the internal medicine, nephrology, ear, nose and throat (ENT) step-down and dermatology inpatient units at Cleveland Clinic main campus. Among her career accomplishments, Simon is most noted for her contributions in the reduction of hospital acquired pressure ulcers and falls. As a result of her educational and monitoring interventions, she has helped reduce pressure ulcer rates in half for the hospital and reduced fall prevalence by approximately 25 percent for one of Cleveland Clinic's medicine units.

Kathleen A. Singleton, MSN, APRN, CNS, CMSRN

Clinical Nurse Specialist, Medical Surgical Services

Kathleen A. Singleton is a clinical nurse specialist in medical-surgical nursing at Cleveland Clinic Fairview Hospital. With a rich and well-rounded nursing career history, Singleton brings four decades of experience to her leadership position. As a well-known resource within the health system, Singleton assists clinical nurses with workload balance, offering them insight, ideas and solutions. She also shares her knowledge with those in leadership positions, encouraging them to work with confidence, commitment and passion, and to seek evidence-based input and collaborative interprofessional decision-making.

Catherine M. Skowronsky, MSN, APRN, ACNS-BC, CMSRN

Clinical Nurse Specialist, Internal Medicine Behavioral Health

Catherine M. Skowronsky is a clinical nurse specialist for inpatient internal medicine at Cleveland Clinic main campus. As part of her role, Skowronsky is highly involved in quality improvement programs at both the nursing unit and health system levels. One of her notable career accomplishments includes the improvement of patient safety through the introduction of a calculator specific to heparin dosing that requires dual sign-off. Additionally, as a means to better care for patients who are unable to follow instructions to maintain personal safety, she was instrumental in the establishment of the first close observation unit in medicine at Cleveland Clinic.

Marian Soat, MSN, APRN, CCNS, CCRN

Clinical Nurse Specialist, Cardiovascular Intensive Care Unit

Marian Soat is a clinical nurse specialist at Cleveland Clinic main campus. She has worked as a CNS in both the cardiovascular and vascular surgery intensive care units at Cleveland Clinic, with a special focus on bringing evidence-based care to the bedside. Throughout Soat's more than three decades in the nursing profession, she spent 24 years as a staff nurse and clinical instructor at various healthcare organizations in Ohio, New York and Washington, including MetroHealth Medical Center in Cleveland, St. Luke's/Roosevelt Hospital Center in New York City and Overlake Hospital Medical Center in Bellevue, Washington.

Deborah L. Solomon, MSN, APRN, ACNS-BC

Clinical Nurse Specialist, Urology and Women's Health

Deborah L. Solomon is a clinical nurse specialist for the women's health, urology and short-stay units at Cleveland Clinic's main campus. Certified in adult health, Solomon's clinical expertise is in women's health and she has many years of experience caring for patients in postpartum, inpatient gynecology and urology. She is the clinical liaison for postpartum, oncology and benign gynecology, as well as benign and malignant urology patients. Solomon has also spent ample time studying the prevention of catheter associated urinary tract infection (which aided in the development of an educational film on the catheter and leg bag), assisted in the writing of a catheter care protocol and helped with physician, nurse and nursing assistant education on the topic.

Jeanne Sorrell, PhD, RN, FAAN

Senior Nurse Researcher, Retired, Office of Research and Innovation

Jeanne Sorrell has received awards for teaching, research and writing and has been published widely in professional journals where she mentors nurse clinicians in developing research that enhances the nursing profession and improves patient outcomes. Her scholarly interests focus on philosophical inquiry, writing across the curriculum, qualitative research and ethical considerations for patients with chronic illness. Her most recent research has focused on ethical concerns of family caregivers of persons with Alzheimer's disease. She has taught qualitative research methods to masters and doctoral students and has supervised over 50 doctoral students in writing dissertations.

Betsy Stovsky, MSN, RN

Manager, Heart and Vascular Institute Resource Information Center

Betsy Stovsky is manager of the Heart & Vascular Institute Resource and Information Center. The center includes a nurse patient call center, which allows patients to communicate with cardiovascular nurses via phone, on-line chat and webmail. The center also produces Heart & Vascular Institute patient education resources for the Cleveland Clinic health system, including written materials, videos, interactive tools and digital media. Stovsky also serves as manager of the Heart & Vascular Institute's website, which has over 14 million visitors each year and includes cardiovascular health and recovery information, online chats and videos.

Anne O. Vanderbilt, MSN, APRN, CNS, CNP

Director of Advanced Practice Nursing, Clinical Nurse Specialist, Geriatrics

Anne O. Vanderbilt is a clinical nurse specialist, adult nurse practitioner and advanced practice nurse manager at Cleveland Clinic main campus. Vanderbilt holds certifications from the American Nurses Credentialing Center in gerontological nursing and as an adult nurse practitioner. Her CNS experience includes both internal medicine and geriatrics. Leading initiatives such as Cleveland Clinic's geriatric resource nurse program, hospital-wide fall minimization program and a multi-disciplinary falls clinic, Vanderbilt is highly skilled in patient care as well as caregiver education and support.

Monica M. Weber, MSN, APRN, CNS-BC, FAHA

Director of Professional Nursing Practice, Magnet Program Manager

Monica M. Weber is director of professional nursing practice for Cleveland Clinic's Stanley Shalom Zielony Institute for Nursing Excellence and Magnet® program manager for Cleveland Clinic main campus. As director of professional nursing practice, Weber manages the integration of nursing policies and procedures, excellence programs and shared governance. Her responsibilities surrounding the Cleveland Clinic main campus Magnet program include providing guidance in the areas of quality patient care, nursing excellence and innovations in nursing practice.

Anita J. White, MSN, APRN, ACNS-BC, CCRN

Clinical Nurse Specialist, Medical Intensive Care Unit

Anita J. White is a clinical nurse specialist for the medical intensive care unit at Cleveland Clinic's main campus. A dedicated member of the American Association of Critical Care Nursing (AACN), White has served the organization as program chair and past-president for the Lake Erie chapter, leading the chapter to receive two national AACN awards. With expertise in chest pain, she has also led the coordination of chest pain center accreditation for three hospitals, producing positive results in all three hospitals and earning gold-level recognition from the American Heart Association for two hospitals.

Erica R. Yates, MSN, APRN, ACNS-BC, CRRN

Clinical Nurse Specialist, Acute Rehabilitation and Epilepsy

Erica R. Yates is a board-certified adult clinical nurse specialist and certified rehabilitation registered nurse at Cleveland Clinic main campus. An expert resource for her colleagues, Yates serves as a clinical leader, incorporating evidence-based practice into the daily care of patients. Yates joined the Cleveland Clinic team in 2011 and shortly after, became a clinical nurse specialist. Previously, she served as a clinical nurse for four years at Cleveland's University Hospitals' Case Medical Center. She currently serves as the NICHE co-coordinator at main campus as well as covering the Acute Rehabilitation unit and the Adult Epilepsy Monitoring Unit.

Amy R. Young, MSN, APRN, ACNS-AG, CCRN

Clinical Nurse Specialist, Neurology Intensive Care and Step-down

Amy R. Young is a clinical nurse specialist in the neurological and neurosurgical intensive care unit and step-down unit at Cleveland Clinic main campus. Her professional experience includes impacting patient care across the inpatient care continuum, mentoring new staff nurses and implementing evidence-based practice within her unit

Index